Iontophoresis in Dental Practice

L. P. Gangarosa, Sr., Ph.D., D.D.S.

Professor of Oral Biology and Pharmacology
Coordinator of Pharmacology for Dentistry
Medical College of Georgia School of Dentistry

quintessence
books

Quintessence Publishing Co., Inc. 1983
Chicago, Berlin, Rio de Janeiro, Tokyo

Lithography: Sun Art Printing, Osaka
Composition: Beslow, Chicago
Printing: Christian Board of Publication, St. Louis
Binding: Becktold Co., St. Louis
Printed in U.S.A

ISBN 0-931386-52-7

Table of Contents

Preface

This monograph addresses itself to a topic which is most timely, namely, the delivery of medications to their site of action. Many medications available today may be under-utilized because they cannot reach the site of action in proper concentrations. Since many medications are ionized, they do not ordinarily penetrate into surface tissue to the extent that their maximum therapeutic effect can be achieved.

This penetration problem of ionic drugs can be largely overcome by providing an energy source which will increase the degree of penetration and thus, the concentration of medication at the desired site of action. Electricity represents a form of energy which can be utilized to assist the movement of various ions to the site of action.

The iontophoresis information presented in this book will provide the practitioner with an excellent understanding of the principles of this valuable mode of therapy. Having established this understanding the book then presents, in clear and adequate detail, the methodology of iontophoresis. I have used the ElectroApplicator System described in this book for the treatment of hypersensitive dentin, which had been treated *unsuccessfully* by all other modes of therapy. The response of my patients to treatment with iontophoresis was most gratifying. The majority obtained complete relief after one treatment and most of the others responded to therapy after a second treatment! For this reason, iontophoresis is now an important part of my practice of periodontics.

This book also discusses the use of iontophoresis in obtaining surface local anesthesia, in the application of anti-inflammatory medications for apthous ulcers and lichen planus and in the management of oral viral lesions.

I believe that the reader will find this book to be most readable and will find the ElectroApplicator System described to be simple to use and most effective in the daily treatment of patients.

Sebastian G. Ciancio, Chairman
Periodontics and Endodontics
SUNY, Buffalo, NY

Acknowledgements

The author wishes to acknowledge the help of Jeff Blankenship, Milt Burroughs, Maria Gangarosa, Louis Hinley, Dorothy M. Lyons, Dwayne T. McGahee, Keith McRae, Barbara M. Peebles, and Dorothy B. Smith who all provided various technical services in the preparation of this manuscript. The author is extremely grateful for the support of Drs. Thomas A. Garman, Gerald A. Heuer, James M. Hill, Arthur Jeske, Byong S. Kwon, Hubert M. Merchant, No Hee Park and Richard E. Walton who aided in development of the techniques presented, in patient care and in research support. The author wishes to express his gratitude to the Medical College of Georgia for providing the atmosphere needed to pursue this work. Many thanks to Dr. Sebastian Ciancio, Chairman, Periodontics and Endodontics, SUNY, Buffalo, NY, who first evaluated the author's specified system in 1974–76 and again in 1980–81 and who wrote the forward to this book. Finally, the author wishes to acknowledge the long-suffering support of his family who sacrificed many hours of companionship so that this work could be possible.

The author dedicates this work to his wife (Clara) and children, (Michael, Louis Jr., Maria and Alyssa). Through their sacrifices, I hope that many dental patients will be relieved of discomfort and many dentists will improve the quality of their practices.

Section I

Basis for Iontophoresis in Dentistry

Chapter 1

Introduction and Rationale

Iontophoresis is a preferred method of applying ions or ionic drugs to surface tissues. When salts are dissolved, ionized or electrically charged, particles are formed in aqueous solution. The process of ion formation is called dissociation or ionization. There are many substances suitable for medication of oral tissues which have a salt or ionic character. Lidocaine hydrochloride, epinephrine hydrochloride, and sodium fluoride are examples of important dental medications which are salts.

Ionized drugs or chemicals do not ordinarily penetrate into surface tissues at a rapid enough rate to achieve a therapeutic level. Surface tissues, such as oral mucosa, consist of membrane barriers which are rich in lipids or fats. Drugs which are lipid-soluble (nonionized) are more readily absorbed by membranes than water-soluble, ionized substances. Thus, if one wishes to achieve surface anesthesia, lidocaine base, dissolved in an ointment or a similar lipid-based vehicle, is applied. On the other hand, drugs for injection into body tissues must be highly water soluble. For injection purposes, the ionized drug is preferred. Lidocaine hydrochloride, the salt form of the drug, is used in injection solutions. If one were to apply lidocaine hydrochloride solution to the mucosa, no surface anesthesia would result because the ionic drug would not penetrate.

Although the lipid-soluble lidocaine base penetrates more readily into oral mucosa than the ionic form, the process of penetration is still slow. It takes several minutes to achieve even a slight anesthetic effect after applying lidocaine ointment to the oral mucosa. The penetration of substances from ointments into tissues is usually slow because the driving force depends upon chemical differences in concentration. The law of diffusion states that the greater the difference in concentration, the greater the rate of penetration. Furthermore, penetration is delayed by a diffusion barrier, oral mucosa or skin, in spite of the lipid nature of both lidocaine base and the surface barrier.

The problem of membrane penetration of ionic drugs can be overcome by providing an energy source which increases the rate of penetration. Electrical energy, in the form of a slight direct current, will assist the movement of ions. According to electrical principles, like charges repel each other and opposite charges attract. Thus, positive ions are repelled from the positive electrode and attracted to the negative electrode. In an analagous manner, negative ions are attracted to the positive electrode and repelled from the negative electrode. In order to electrically assist the introduction of the positively charged lidocaine into oral mucosa, the drug must be applied under a positively charged electrode (anode). The penetration of the neg-

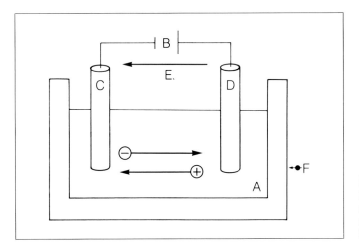

Fig. 1 Movement of ions in solution: a) solution, b) battery, c) cathode (−), d) anode (+), e) direction of electron flow, f) beaker.

atively charged fluoride ion can be assisted by applying fluoride under a negative electrode (cathode).

The diagram in Figure 1 indicates how ions move in an electrolyte solution (A). When a DC voltage is applied by a battery (B), positively charged ions (called cations) are attracted to the cathode (C) and repelled from the anode (D). Likewise, negatively charged ions (called anions) are attracted to the anode and repelled from the cathode. The transport of electrical current occurs in solution by the movement of ions; however, in an electrical wire circuit, only negative particles (electrons) can move, as indicated by the arrow (E) (Fig. 1).

Let us consider what happens in a patient, when iontophoresis is performed (Fig. 2). The active electrode* is placed over the tissues which require medication, e.g. a lesion on the skin. The indifferent or return electrode* is placed at a convenient location anywhere on the body, for example

the arm (B). The two electrodes are connected to a direct current source, (C), either a battery or a D.C. rectifier. If a negatively charged drug is to be introduced, the medicating-solution is placed under the negative electrode (cathode), and the return electrode, containing an indifferent electrolyte (such as, sodium nitrate or any other salt solution) is placed at another convenient area of the body. The current is then gradually increased until the patient feels a slight sensation. The electrical energy causes the negatively charged drug to enter the surface tissues contacting the negative electrode.

Once the drug enters the tissue, it does not follow the pathway through the patient to the return electrode; rather, chloride ions (the principle extracellular anions) carry the current to the other electrode by following the pathway of least resistance in the body. Just as in the case of current traveling in the electrolyte, the positive ions (sodium) move from positive to negative electrode, in the path of least resistance. If the medicating substance is positive, the electrodes are reversed; the active electrode becomes the positive

---

* In this text "active electrode" is synonymous with "treatment electrode" and "return (indifferent) electrode" is synonymous with "dispersive electrode."

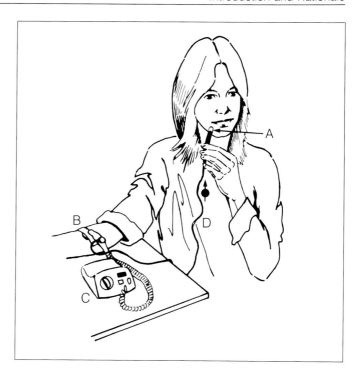

Fig. 2 Set-up for iontophoresis in a patient: a) area of lesion, b) area of placement of indifferent electrode, c) iontophoretic power source, d) direction of electron flow.

electrode and the indifferent electrode is negative. As in any electrical wire circuit, electrons complete the path by traveling in the direction indicated by the arrow (D).

Diagramatically, we may view the set-up for application of drugs by iontophoresis as in Figures 3 and 4. A power supply (A) contains a DC source, a milliammeter (B) a rheostat (C), which sets the external voltage bias, and two electrodes, one positive and one negative. In Figure 3, the set-up for delivering a positive drug is shown. As an example, lidocaine HCl is placed under the positive electrode which forces positive ions into the adjacent tissue. Negative ions are forced in the opposite direction at the positive electrode. At the negative electrode an indifferent electrolyte, such as sodium nitrate, is placed and negative nitrate ions enter, while positive sodium ions are forced in the opposite direction.

Figure 4 shows the set-up for delivery of a negative drug, such as fluoride and the explanation is similar to that provided for Figure 3, except that fluoride ion is delivered at the negative electrode and the indifferent solution is placed at the positive electrode. In both cases, the extracellular cation (sodium) and anion (chloride) complete the circuit, in the extracellular fluid, by following the pathway of least resistance (D).

This brief introduction indicates why iontophoresis is the method of choice for application of ionic drugs to surface tissues. Although lipid-soluble bases of drugs penetrate surface tissues more rapidly than ionized drugs when diffusion is used as the driving force for penetration, iontophoresis of the ionic form of the drug offers a distinct advantage over diffusion of either the base or the ionic form.

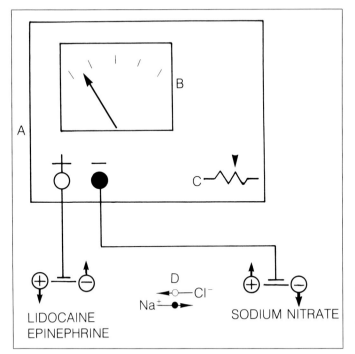

Fig. 3 Set-up for delivery of positive drugs: a) Power source, b) Milliammeter, c) Rheostat, d) Direction of current (ion) flow.

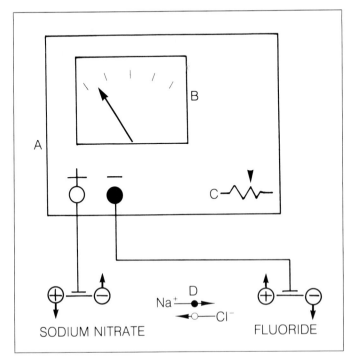

Fig. 4 Set-up for delivery of negative drugs: a) Power source, b) Milliammeter, c) Rheostat, d) Direction of current (ion) flow.

Chapter 2

History of Use of Iontophoresis in Medicine and Dentistry

Medicine

The process of introducing ions for therapeutic purposes was first attempted in 1841, for delivery of mercury and iodine into body tissues.[96] After the discovery of cocaine's anesthetic effect in 1864,[32] cocaine iontophoresis was utilized in several specialities.[2] In 1896, Morton reported on the cocaine "cataphoresis" of the dental pulp. LeDuc[57] reviewed the status of iontophoresis about the turn of the century, and he attempted to explain the process in physicochemical terms.

In the first half of the 1900's, many uses of iontophoresis were attempted; the subject was reviewed by Abramowitsch and Neoussikine,[2] who listed many indications for iontophoresis in medicine, and by Harris.[40] The latter author described the following uses: 1) heavy metal iontophoresis (Zn for antibacterial effect, Cu as a fungicide, Ag for osteoarthritis); 2) for vasodilation (histamine or methacholine); 3) for vasoconstriction (epinephrine); 4) for local anesthesia of the skin (procaine or dibucaine with epinephrine); 5) in scleroderma or lymphedema (hyaluronidase); 6) in rheumatoid arthritis (citrate); 7) in corneal ulcers (Zn); and 8) for hyperhydrosis (constant current application).

Gibson and Cooke[31] advocated an iontophoretic method of pilocarpine introduction into skin in order to produce sweating. The sweat obtained was analyzed for sodium and chloride and the data used for cystic fibrosis diagnosis. As a result, the pilocarpine iontophoresis is well accepted, and is used many times daily in most major medical centers, throughout the USA, to diagnose cystic fibrosis in infants and children.

Iontophoresis of vasodilators for peripheral vascular diseases was recommended by Stone,[93] although this use appears to be limited in popularity.

Comeau et al.[11] reported that anesthesia of the eardrum could be obtained by lidocaine and epinephrine iontophoresis. This technique has been well accepted in ENT practice; the Editor of *Eye, Ear, Nose and Throat*[45] called lidocaine-epinephrine iontophoresis, "A major advancement for myringotomy and ear drum surgery." Gangarosa[16] reported on lidocaine-epinephrine iontophoresis for oral mucosal anesthesia, but he used a much lower concentration of epinephrine (20-40 μg/ml) compared to Comeau (500 μg/ml). Sisler[90] reported that corneal surgery could be performed after lidocaine-epinephrine iontophoresis using a modification of the Comeau-Vernon technique. A recent article in Med. News & Int. Rep.[47] indicates that anesthesia of the skin for artificial kidney dialysis cut-down was successful. It appears that surface anesthesia of any surface of the body can be obtained using lidocaine-epinephrine iontophoresis, and that the technique is currently accepted for certain uses in medical practice.

A well established use of iontophoresis is the treatment of hyperhydrosis of the palms and soles. Shelley et al.[85] reasoned that, since iontophoresis of many substances had been used successfully to treat hyperhydrosis (including aluminum chloride, potassium permanganate and formaldehyde), the beneficial inhibition of sweating was probably caused by constant current application. Therefore, they used tap water iontophoresis and found an improvement in 90% of patients. Research reports which verify the anhydrotic effect of iontophoresis include: Shelley et al.[85] Shelley and Horvath,[86] Grice and Bettley,[37] Levit,[61] Gordon and Maibach,[33] Grice, Satter, and Baker,[38] Abell and Morgan,[1] and Shrivastava and Singh.[87]

Iontophoresis of antimicrobial agents has been reported. Von Sallmann[94] reported that sulfadiazine iontophoresis caused a high concentration of the drug in the aqueous humor, while having a beneficial effect in rabbits and humans with pyocyaneous keratitis of the eye. Von Sallmann[95] reported that penicillin iontophoresis would produce high concentrations of the drug in rabbit eyes, although the results were less favorable in normal or edematous human eyes. Witzel et al.[98] reported that iontophoresis favorably increased penetration of streptomycin, dihydrostreptomycin and neomycin into rabbit eyes; iontophoresis equalled other methods which produced high concentrations of penicillin, magnamycin and erythromycin, while it was of no value for polymyxin B, bacitracin and tetracycline. Fellner and Glawogger[15] studied penicillin levels in aqueous and vitreous humors of human eyes and concluded that iontophoresis was "valuable reinforcement of local therapy." Jenkinson and McLean[48] reported

successful results with iontophoresis of methylene blue (demodex in dogs) and potassium iodide (fungal infection of cattle). LaForest and Cofrancesco[56] reported successful treatment of suppurative ear chondritis by gentamycin iontophoresis.

Recently Greminger et al.[36] confirmed the latter work by reporting on 11 more successful treatments using gentamycin iontophoresis for ear chondritis after burns or plastic procedures.

The subject of antiviral chemotherapy by iontophoresis was investigated by Gangarosa and his colleagues.[18-21,23,28,29] They treated herpesvirus infections by idoxuridine iontophoresis in a limited number of human volunteers with orofacial herpes labialis to demonstrate effectiveness of the technique[28,29] the results were dramatic, with early resolution of the lesions. Further, they showed that idoxuridine[19] and the newer antiviral drug, ara-AMP (adenine arabinoside monophosphate) would concentrate in skin[20] when the drugs were applied by iontophoresis. Also, they showed that the antiviral drugs applied by iontophoresis to mouse skin would inhibit DNA synthesis[19-21] and effectively counteract viral infections of mouse skin.[23,29]

In addition, iontophoresis of drugs has been reported to be useful for the following conditions: (see chart).

The author does not consider that all these claims are proven. In fact, there are no controlled studies supporting these uses. A great deal of research needs to be done before such uses are acceptable in medical practice.

In summary, from a review of the literature, one can conclude that there are several valid uses of iontophoresis in medicine, including, pilocarpine for cystic fibrosis diagnosis, local anesthetics for minor surgery of surface tissues, epinephrine for vasoconstriction as an aid to local anesthesia and sodium chloride iontophoresis

Condition	Drug Used	Author and Year
Tumors and cancers	general review	Peterson & Strelkova, 1964
	bleomycin	Hayasaki, et al, 1977
Peyronies Disease	glucocorticoids	Rothfeld & Murray, 1967
Vasomotor nasal disorders	Zn	Weir, 1967
Plantar warts	sodium salicylate	Gordon & Weinstein, 1969
Soft tissue hemorrhage	hyaluronidase	Boone, 1969
Vitiligo	melanidine	Moawad, 1969
Myopathy	calcium	Kahn, 1975
Calcium deposits	acetic acid	Kahn, 1977

for hyperhydrosis. In addition, there are *no* effective and acceptable treatments available for virus infections of skin; iontophoresis offers the hope that assistance of penetration of antiviral drugs will be an effective means of therapy. The use of iontophoresis in other types of medical therapy needs to be thoroughly investigated before the claims are accepted.

Dentistry

Iontophoresis has had a long history of use in dentistry. As was mentioned earlier, Morton[70] was one of the first to report on cocaine iontophoresis, using it for anesthesia of the dental pulp. The early history of use in dentistry was reviewed by Abramowitsch and Neoussikine.[2] In 1931, Grossman reported that sterilization of root canals could be facilitated by electrolysis. Siemon[88] and Manning[65] were responsible for introducing fluoride iontophoresis for dentin desensitization into the U.S.A. following reports on the subject by Japanese workers.[53,54] Many reports on fluoride iontophoresis of dentin followed (see reviews: Murthy et al.[71]; Gangarosa and Park[24]). Gangarosa[16] reported on iontophoretic introduction of local anesthetics and epi-

nephrine into oral mucosa producing a profound surface anesthesia, sufficient to extract loose deciduous teeth. Gangarosa and co-workers[28] reported that idoxuridine iontophoresis was effective in treating herpes labialis.

A group of Italian odontologists have recently presented many papers, which were summarized in a monograph on iontophoresis entitled "Manual of Iontophoresis in the Oral Cavity (Electrical Application of Drugs in Stomatology)", by A. Benedicenti and L. Cingano.[5] This work was rather obscure to the author and only became available for translation recently when the author made a trip to Genoa to present his results on use of iontophoresis in dentistry in the U.S. The Italian group presented studies on a wide variety of chemicals which have varied pharmacological activities. Their monograph described the apparatus used in Italy and how the direction of movement (from cathode to anode or vice versa) was determined using electrophoretic laboratory procedures. They also presented numerable uses in both dentistry and medicine with the drug protocols and electrical parameters used for treating each condition. Generally, the author feels that many more documentations of the Italian studies are needed. They tend to use much more current (mA) and frequency of retreatment than used by the author in the U.S.

The author's experience with iontophoresis supports the following uses of this technique in dental practice: 1) fluoride treatment of exposed hypersensitive dentin, 2) steroid iontophoresis of aphthous ulcers and other inflammatory conditions, 3) idoxuridine iontophoresis of herpes labialis and 4) lidocaine-epinephrine iontophoresis for local anesthesia of oral mucosa. Each of these subjects will be considered in detail in subsequent sections of this monograph. The subject of electrolysis of pulp canals for sterilization will not be considered here because it is beyond the scope of this monograph.

Chapter 3

Rationale for Treating Hypersensitive Teeth

Many dental patients have exposed hypersensitive dentin. There are many causes of exposure of the dentin including erosion, abrasion, hypoplastic enamel, improperly formed cemento-enamel junctions, occlusal wear, caries, cracking, trauma and iatrogenic. The latter, i.e. induction of dentin exposure by the dentist, is particularly bothersome to both patient and dentist; it occurs as a result of therapy for periodontal disease, in tooth restoration, in occlusal equilibration, etc.

The dentist has a number of methods of coping with exposed dentin. In the case of caries or trauma, the tooth may be restored. Onlays or overlay dentures may be appropriate for massive occlusal wear. Many dentists and periodontists believe that good plaque control is important to prevent further erosive action of chemicals formed in plaque. Cracked teeth or those with irreversible pulp changes may be treated by standard endodontic therapy.

The dentist may use "desensitizing medicaments" or recommend a "desensitizing" toothpaste for home use. Although indicated restorative or endodontic treatments may be very effective in treating some causes of dentin exposure, in most other cases, the treatment of hypersensitive dentin has been rather ineffective. The "desensitizing medicaments" are often caustic, sometimes causing discoloration, and may be no more effective than placebos. The "desensitizing toothpastes," although convenient, have often been disappointing, and usually show effects equivalent to, or only slightly better than, placebos.[71]

It would be helpful in dentistry to have available an effective, biologically safe method for treating painful, hypersensitive exposed dentin. This would relieve many patients of discomfort which can be bothersome and often severe. Many patients are unable to eat in comfort and some suffer from the mere passage of air through the mouth, as in breathing or speaking. Such discomfort often follows periodontal surgery and reconstructive dentistry, where large areas of dentin are exposed. Often the patient becomes so sensitive that drilling and other necessary procedures become difficult for the dentist, slowing completion of the case. When this happens to a reconstruction case, or following one quadrant of periodontal surgery, the patient may be reluctant or unwilling to allow the dentist to complete the treatment.

The dentist therefore needs a treatment for dentin desensitization which is close to "ideal." Grossman[39] suggested that the ideal desensitizer: (1) should not be unduly irritating to the pulp, (2) should be relatively painless, (3) should be easy to apply, (4) should be consistently and permanently effective, (5) should act quickly, and (6) should not cause tooth discoloration. The agents currently in use should be evaluated according to these criteria. Since caustic agents irritate the pulp, they should not be placed on exposed dentin.[84] This would eliminate silver nitrate, zinc chloride, phenol, formaldehyde, concentrated alcohols, acids or alkalis. Some dentists currently recommend calcium hydroxide pastes, but the high pH of such preparations may be irritating and result in pulpal damage.

Topical fluoride therapy does appear to be promising as a method of tooth desensitization. Lukomsky[63] suggested that sodium fluoride applied to dentin forms an effective surface barrier and results in desensitization of dentin. He described his methods of application, but gave no experimental details or quantitative results. Hoyt and Bibby[43] used a paste, suggested by Lukomsky, which contained equal parts of sodium fluoride, clay and glycerin; desensitization occurred in approximately 80% of the treatments. Their study did not include controls, and they did not adequately describe their method of evaluation. It should be mentioned that the following research reports implicate high concentrations of fluoride as irritating to the odontoblasts: Lefkowitz and Bodecker;[58] Rovelstad and St. John;[81] Maurice and Schour;[66] and Brännström and Nyborg.[7]

Many fluoride salts have been reported to be effective in reducing dentin hypersensitivity when applied as dentifrices or as topical agents (Murthy et al[71]). Such studies indicate that various sources of fluoride have some degree of efficacy implicating fluoride as the active agent.

Many of our patients at the Medical College of Georgia, School of Dentistry, have received treatment with the 33.3% sodium fluoride paste and/or have used fluoride-containing dentifrices. Other patients have used a strontium chloride dentifrice that has been reported by Ross,[79] Meffert and Hoskins,[67] and Pusso-Carrasco[78] and others to be effective in desensitization. Since most of our patients have continued to complain of intolerable discomfort after such treatments, a method of assuring fluoride penetration into the dentinal tubules suggested itself as a means of enhancing desensitization of dentin. Since iontophoresis appears to be an ideal method for enhancement of penetration of ions into surface tissues, the use of the fluoride iontophoresis appears to have a rational basis for aiding fluoride penetration into dentin.

Iontophoresis of fluoride has been suggested as a method of treating hypersensitive dentin since the mid 1950's.[53,54] Siemon[88] and Manning[65] described the use of battery-operated devices* to apply current to teeth, and a brush electrode to aid fluoride penetration into dentin; the indifferent (return) electrode was hand-held. Siemon[88] claimed 85% effectiveness, but his data were based on only a small number of patients. Manning[65] claimed that his method was effective in eliminating pain from cold-air blasts on exposed cervical dentin, but his report presented no data. Eshleman and Leonard[14] reviewed the literature and described their clinical observations using the method of Siemon on 32 patients. They claimed that there was immediate, long-term (12 to 19 months), and extremely effective reduction of sensitivity. No data were presented and no controls were described. Schaeffer and associates[82] used an iontophoretic toothbrush and a stannous fluoride dentifrice. They claimed that all patients who received electrical current, with or without fluoride, experienced desensitization. However, the

---

*Chayes Dental Instrument Corp., Danbury, CT, Lemos Co., Miami, FL.

toothbrush that they used delivered a positive charge to the teeth. Since the positive charge opposes the penetration of fluoride, any beneficial effects observed by Schaeffer may have been due to other factors than fluoride iontophoresis.

Collins[10] noted that chair-side desensitization had only a transient effect and that home supplementation by means of an ionizing toothbrush** was required to eliminate or reduce sensitivity. His study was double-blind in that control patients also received toothbrushes, but the batteries had been removed. He reported an 85% reduction in dentin sensitivity of the experimental group, but only about a 20% reduction for the control group. In agreement with the studies of Collins, Jensen[49] reported on the ionizing toothbrush; the experimental group showed at least a 75% reduction in sensitivity, while 10% was the highest reduction in control patients.

Scott[83] also presented a review of the literature on fluoride iontophoresis and attempted to determine whether current would damage the odontoblasts. He applied current to freshly cut dentin and concluded that 1 milliampere of electricity applied for 1 minute (1 mA-min) caused no permanent injury. He claimed that desensitization occurred without lowering pulp vitality when this limit was observed.

Lefkowitz[59] and Lefkowitz and associates[60] were interested in pulp response and the mechanism of desensitization following iontophoresis of sound human teeth that had been indicated for extraction for prosthetic reasons. After they prepared Class V cavities having remaining dentin 1.2 mm thick, the experimenters applied the negative electrode into the cavity using either sodium fluoride, or the patient's saliva, as the electrolyte. They claimed that the cur-

rent induced rapid formation of massive reparative dentin within 7-28 days, without causing permanent pulpal damage, whether sodium fluoride or saliva was applied. The studies of Leftkowitz need to be repeated because recent studies of reparative dentin formation[92] indicate that reparative dentin formation occurs at a much slower rate than reported by Lefkowitz.

Murthy and associates[71] used a sable-brush applicator attached to a direct-current source for the iontophoresis of sodium fluoride and of saliva. Topical treatment with 33.3% sodium fluoride was also evaluated. This excellent study reported on an adequate number of subjects and used a double-blind procedure, the correct negative charge and an appropriate, subjective evaluation. The authors concluded that sodium fluoride iontophoresis provided the most effective treatment and that the desensitization was immediate in most patients.

Minkov and associates[68] also used an adequate number of subjects and appropriate evaluation procedures, but they concluded that 2% sodium fluoride applied topically, either with or without current (2 treatments per week for 6 weeks), was effective in desensitizing dentin. However, like Schaeffer and associates (see above), they used a positive electrode on the tooth.

Summary of the Earlier Literature

About 1975, many studies had recommended the fluoride iontophoresis for desensitization. Since iontophoresis assists penetration of ions into tissues, there is rational basis for using an electrical current to carry fluoride into the tooth. Many clinical observations indicate the effectiveness of fluoride iontophoresis, but only one study[71] proved effectiveness and was ad-

**The Ion Toothbrush, The Ion Co., Los Angeles, CA.

equately controlled and properly conducted. Two groups that did not demonstrate the effectiveness of fluoride iontophoresis used the wrong polarity on the tooth electrode: one claimed the current alone was effective[82] and the other[68] claimed that the fluoride was effective with or without current.[68] The studies on the iontophoretic toothbrush[10,49] are generally supportive of fluoride iontophoresis. Nevertheless, over the years, iontophoretic toothbrushing has not gained acceptance among dentists or patients for various reasons. One problem involves the present design of the electrode placement which favors current flow through saliva rather than into the tooth.[89]

Development of Modern Iontophoresis

Our studies on desensitization of dentin, at the Medical College of Georgia, started about 1972 as a result of the author's interest in local anesthesia and pain control. We had been studying iontophoretic application of local anesthetics to the skin even before that time. We had developed the philosophy that any drug of choice could be better delivered to a body surface by iontophoresis than by any other method of application. Since the literature indicated that fluoride was an effective agent for hypersensitive dentin, and others had tried iontophoresis to assist penetration, We then analyzed the problem, "Why hasn't fluoride iontophoresis gained wide acceptance?" It soon became apparent that a new technique was needed because the equipment available at that time (1972) was crude and the methods used were poorly conceived.

The problems with fluoride iontophoretic technology involved 1) an inadequate power supply, 2) no insulation provided, and 3) poor adaptation of electrodes to the teeth. We therefore concentrated on developing a new system for fluoride iontophoresis which provides: 1) an adequate power supply, 2) a flexible electrode system which adapts to all areas of the dentition, and 3) insulation. We also gave much thought to safety and prescribed the amounts of current which would provide a safe, biologically acceptable technique, with no pulpal damage.

Our initial studies, started in 1972, were reported in two publications in 1978.[24,25] Methods used are demonstrated in Figures 5–7. Figure 5a shows the indifferent electrode (left) plugged into the positive terminal and the active electrode plugged into the negative terminal, for fluoride delivery. The power unit (ElectroApplicator™ Model C-1) contains (left to right) a milliammeter, an off-on current switch which also increases the voltage bias, and a timer. On the lower part of the instrument panel, there are (left to right) the electrode terminals, a charge outlet (for recharging Nicad batteries) and a timer on-off switch. In the upper center, a pilot light indicated that the unit was operational.

Although this power supply unit was a great stride forward from the technology available in the early 1970's, several newer features have been introduced in a more advanced design (Model C-2) which will be discussed in Section III of this monograph. The electrode leads, needed to perform dependable iontophoresis, are shown in Figure 5b. Starting with upper left, row one, there are alligator clip electrodes, an empty space, and alcohol swabs to wipe the skin. The second row contains different sizes of plastic tips, for adaptation to the teeth. The third row contains the skin electrodes, brush electrodes, and skin electrode pads. In the fourth row are oral electrodes and a strap for the skin electrode. The fifth row contains leads for the return (skin) electrode

Figs. 5a and 5b Electro-Applicator, model C-1 (EA, C-1).

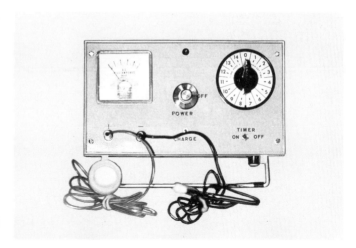

Fig. 5a Power source and electrodes.

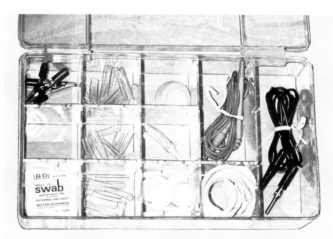

Fig. 5b Electrode set.

or for the alligator clips. (More details on these parts are found later in Section III of this monograph; many new features have been incorporated into the Dentelect Electrode Set™, by LPG.) All items are color-coded; red indicates positive and black, negative.

Figure 6a shows a close-up of the return (skin) electrode attached to a patient's arm. For fluoride iontophoresis, the return (also called indifferent) electrode, is red and is attached to the positive pole of the power supply. Figure 6b shows a close-up of the configuration of return electrode used previously. A disposable electrode pad is placed in a nylon ring containing a wire mesh. The pad is soaked with 1% sodium nitrate, and a banana plug is inserted into the opposite side of the nylon; metal to metal contact is made between wire mesh and banana plug.

Figure 7a shows the completely assembled oral electrode. The exploded view in Figure 7b shows how the oral electrode is assembled. The oral electrode is a flexible plastic probe which can be bent to any an-

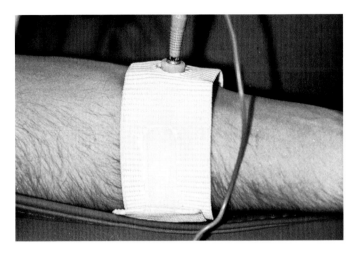

Figs. 6a and 6b   Return electrode, EA, C-1.

Fig. 6a   Complete set-up.

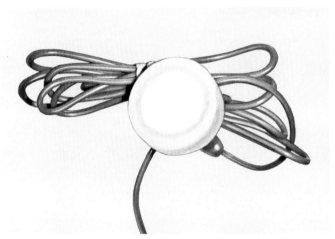

Fig. 6b   Area which contacts skin.

gle for ease in reaching inaccessible areas of the mouth. The plastic tips come in several sizes and can be contoured to fit the facial area of various teeth. The plastic tip fits over the oral electrode, leaving room for cotton to contact the metal. A single wisp of cotton is placed in the opening; the cotton is soaked with 2% sodium fluoride and must make intimate contact with the dentin lesion, as well as the metal tip of the oral electrode.

Figure 8 shows how the oral electrode is applied to the tooth for the usual case of cervical hypersensitivity. Figure 8a shows the rubber dam in place, and the plastic tip occluding the dentin lesion. Although this placement may seem ideal, it was found that the rubber dam often interferes with close contact to the dentin lesion. Equally effective desensitization can be obtained by placing an appropriate, sized and contoured, plastic tip over the tooth; this retracts the gingiva and acts as an insulator, preventing loss of current (Fig. 8b). Two other configurations of the electrode system are: 1) a brush, for interproximal

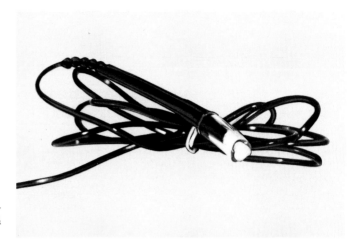

Fig. 7a   Oral electrode, Electro-Applicator system (EAS, C-2 & EA, C-1) assembled.

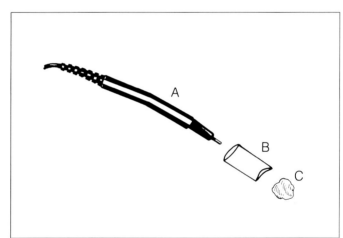

Fig. 7b   Exploded view: a) oral electrode, b) plastic tip, c) Cotton (for Drug).

sensitivity or for areas where insulation is not obtainable, and 2) a clip, for the tray technique of treating multiple hypersensitivities. These modifications will be discussed, for latest techniques of desensitization in use, in Chapter 13.

Continuing with methods from our 1978 reports, the circuit was completed as indicated in Figures 6a and 8. The power unit switch was turned to ON and the current slowly increased, either to a preset maximum of 0.5 mA (for one tooth), or until the patient first feels a slight, tingling sensa-tion in the tooth, whichever is less. A dose of one mA-min was delivered to each tooth. Sensitivity was evaluated by a standardized, one-second blast of air directed at each sensitive tooth, both before and after treatment, with the surrounding teeth insulated. The patient was asked to rate the sensitivity on the following subjective discomfort scale: 0 = normal sensation; 1 = mild discomfort; 2 = moderate; 3 = transient, severe; and 4 = intolerable (severe and lasting beyond the period of stimulus application).

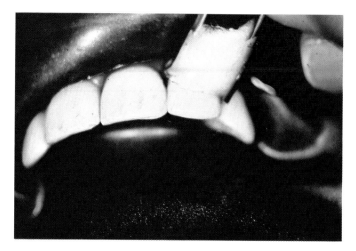

Figs. 8a and 8b Oral electrode set-up (EAS, C-2 and EA, C-1).

Fig. 8a With rubber dam isolation.

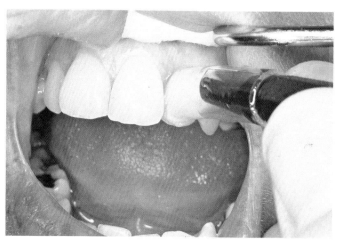

Fig. 8b With cotton roll isolation.

The results of the first study[24] are summarized in Table 1. Increased sensitivity was found when sodium chloride was the electrolyte and the negative electrode was applied to the tooth. This was noted when we attempted to develop the sodium chloride iontophoresis as an electrical control; the procedure was not repeated further because it was extremely distressing to the patients. Under a positive electrode, 2% sodium fluoride provided a moderate reduction of sensitivity in four out of five teeth, while in one tooth it provided a good reduction. When fluoride iontophoresis was used under the proper negative electrode, the results obtained on dentin sensitivity caused by exposed cervical dentin, cavity preparation, hypoplastic enamel, or occlusal wear were dramatic. There was immediate relief of long duration. Reduced sensitivity lasted for the duration of the experiment, which was at least 3 months and up to 3 years, for ten of the patients.

In trials on root dentin exposed following periodontal surgery, there was a good reduction in 64% of the trials and moderate

Table 1 Clinical Trials of Dentin Desensitization by Iontophoresis[a]

Trial	No. patients/ no. teeth	Electrode	Immediate effect on sensitivity[b]
1% sodium chloride for cervical dentin exposure	3/3	Cathode(−)	More sensitive (100%)
2% sodium fluoride:			
1. Reverse polarity for cervical dentin exposure	5/5	Anode(+)	Moderate reduction (80%) Good reduction (20%)
2. Cervical dentin exposure	9/41	Cathode	Good reduction (100%)
3. Inlay or crown preparations	4/17	Cathode	Good reduction (100%)
4. After periodontal surgery	4/25	Cathode	Moderate reduction (36%) Good reduction (64%)
5. Hypoplastic enamel	1/2	Cathode	Good reduction (100%)
6. Occlusal wear	2/21	Cathode	Good reduction (100%)

[a]Results of Gangarosa and Park (1978a)
[b]Effect: Good reduction—complete relief, no retreatment needed.
Moderate reduction—relief, but not complete or retreatment needed to obtain complete relief.
No improvement
More sensitive

reduction in 36%. In the nine teeth having sensitivity reduction rated as moderate, retreatment was required for three teeth after 6 weeks and six teeth after 1 year. The other 16 teeth in that group did not require retreatment for the duration of the experiment. There were no apparent adverse effects of the procedure; the teeth remained healthy and asymptomatic as long as the patients were under observation. Most of these patients have now been under observation for eight years. The treated teeth have vital pulps (by electrical test) and have generally had no return of sensitivity. The results of the second study[25] are shown in Table 2. There were four patients, in this study, with 32 hypersensitive teeth treated by four dental students under the direction of Dr. Gerald Heuer, Associate Professor of Dental Practice Dynamics, Medical College of Georgia. Before the treatment, all teeth rated 2-4 on the discomfort scale (Table 2). After treatment, the discomfort rating was improved in all teeth with 69% of the teeth rated "good improvement" (no remaining discomfort) and

Table 2 Clinical Trials of Dentin Sensitivity (Study 2)

Patient#	Tooth#	Sensitivity[1] Before[2]	After	Improvement[3]
1	5	2	0	G
	11	2	0	G
	20	2	0	G
	21	2	0	G
	29	2	0	G
2	3	4	0	G
	4	4	0	G
	5	4	0	G
	27	4	0	G
	28	4	0	G
	29	4	2	M
	2	4	0	G
	11	4	0	G
	12	4	0	G
	13	4	0	G
3	26	3	1	M
	27	3	2	M
	4	3	1	M
	12	4	0	G
4	20	2	1	M
	22	2	0	G
	23	2	0	G
	24	3	1	M
	25	3	0	G
	26	3	1	M
	27	2	1	M
	28	2	0	G
	6	3	1	M
	8	2	0	G
	9	3	0	G
	10	3	1	M
	11	3	0	G

[1]Sensitivity was rated on a discomfort scale: 0 = normal sensation 3 = severe (transient)
1 = mild discomfort 4 = severe (intolerable)
2 = moderate

[2]All teeth treated had exposed cervical dentin and a rating of 2 or higher on the discomfort scale.

[3]Improvement scale: G = intolerable (4), severe (3) or moderate (2) discomfort before treatment; normal sensation (0) after.
M = improvement but some discomfort remaining.
O = no improvement.

Table 3 Effect of Iontophoresis of NaF on Hypersensitive Teeth

Degree of sensitivity	Before treatment (# of teeth)	After treatment (# of teeth)
0	0	13
1	5	5
2	2	11
3	12	0
4	9	0

The data were obtained from twenty-nine (29) teeth of thirteen (13) patients.
The degree of sensitivity was evaluated by blowing cold air on the sensitive areas (see footnote 1, Table 2).

the other 31% "moderate improvement." Subsequently, the teeth showing moderate improvement were retreated (at a second appointment) after which all teeth rated *one* (mild discomfort) or *zero*. Reasons for not having a perfect result (all teeth rated G after one treatment) may include: current loss through adjacent tissues or restorations, saliva contamination of the cotton applicator (which should be soaked with fluoride solution only), failure of the applicator to cover or adapt to the entire surface of the exposed dentinal lesion, or variability due to other factors (related to lesion type or the patient).

A third study has not been reported except at a Table Clinic. A dental student (B. Nalley), working with dental auxiliaries under the direction of Dr. Heuer, performed treatment on 13 patients, with 29 sensitive teeth. The results are reported in Table 3. It should be noted in the table that before treatment most teeth were rated 3 or 4, while after treatment there was a shift of rating to 0, 1 or 2. In this study, it was noted that ratings of all teeth could be reduced to zero or one with a second or third treatment; retreatments were spaced one week apart (data not shown). This was the basis of our current recommendation that dentists forewarn patients of a possible need for three treatments. However, past and present experience indicate that, one treatment is usually sufficient, two treatments are occasionally needed, and three treatments are rarely needed.

The results of all three studies demonstrate the usefulness of this new iontophoretic technique in dentistry. An immediate and profound desensitization results after using this technique; the results are permanent and cause no adverse reaction. The techniques are simple, rapid and can be easily learned by dental students and dentists. Dental hygienists and auxiliaries can aid in the procedure, considerably reducing the dentist's patient-contact time. These techniques are currently being taught to dental students at the Medical College of Georgia, Loma Linda University, University of Texas Dental Branch (Houston) and SUNY at Buffalo. Continuing Education courses on Iontophoresis in Dental Practice have been given at the Medical College of Georgia, Loma Linda University, University of Texas Dental Branch (Houston), SUNY at Buffalo, Temple University, The University of Tennessee, Washington University at St. Louis and other schools.

In addition, this new iontophoretic technique has been independently evaluated in the Departments of Periodontics at SUNY (Buffalo), Temple University, University of Mississippi and Southern Illinois University. All of the preliminary results of independent evaluation, to date, have been favorable.

The details of this technique for tooth desensitization will be described in the Operating Instruction in Section III of this monograph under "Instruction for Treating Hypersensitive Teeth." Iontophoresis by this technique is useful for all types of dentin sensitivity and will be a valuable addition to the dentist's armamentarium.

Mechanism of Fluoride Desensitization

Since the mechanism of fluoride desensitization of dentin is of interest, the subject will be discussed at this point. Although the exact mechanism by which fluoride iontophoresis produces desensitization of dentin is not known, several hypotheses have been proposed. One mechanism proposed by Lefkowitz and associates[60] involves the formation of reparative dentin following application of current to dentin, which results in dead tracts in the primary dentin. The dead tracts could possibly inhibit the passage of stimuli from the exposed dentin to the pulp. Walton and associates[17,30] applied 2% sodium fluoride or sodium chloride to exposed dentin in dogs by cathodal iontophoresis using current dosages (mA-min) of 1.0 and 5 mA-min. They reported no changes in the architecture of the odontoblasts after 7 or 80 days. These results will be discussed further in Chapter 9. The results obtained by Walton et al. are in agreement with the statement by Scott[83] that the application of a controlled amount of current to the dentin is safe. However,

there was no evidence of formation of secondary or reparative dentin in the dog, even after 80 days. There is need for further research on this mechanism since the results in dogs were not the same as those reported in human teeth by Lefkowitz's group.

A second possible explanation of iontophoretic dentin desensitization is that the electrical current produces parethesia by altering the sensory mechanisms of pain conduction. Gangarosa et al.[22] reported that 5 to 15 μamp or more of direct current blocks conduction in the isolated frog nerve, but the effect is readily reversible. It seems reasonable that the 300 to 500 μamp of current used in desensitization would block dentinal pain conduction, if it is assumed that electrical conduction similar to that observed in nerves is involved in dentin sensation. However, iontophoretic desensitization has a rather long duration so that either the paresthesia is enduring (in contrast to the transient effect on nerves in vitro) or another mechanism having a long-term effect is also active.

A third possible explanation of iontophoretic desensitization is that the concentration of fluoride ions in dentinal tubules may be increased due to the fluoride iontophoresis. This could cause microprecipitation of calcium fluoride that may act to block hydrodynamically-mediated, pain-inducing stimuli. Ehrlich and associates[13] observed increased fluoride uptake in exposed root dentin and precipitations in peritubular dentin after one topical application of 2% sodium fluoride. Souder and Schoonover[91] demonstrated that fluoride and calcium will remineralize dentin. The increased fluoride penetration into dentinal tubules presumably caused by iontophoresis may cause calcium fluoride precipitation, which in turn may decrease fluid movement induced by stimuli.

Recently, in our laboratories we (Wilson et

al)[98] presented evidence which supports this hypothesis and may explain the necessity for the electrical current for effective desensitization. Dr. Wilson was able to analyze 4 micron etches of exposed dentin in extracted human teeth. The surface etch of iontophoretically treated teeth contained 2-4 times more fluoride than topically treated teeth and 24 to 30 times more than control teeth. In the fourth etch, iontophoresis raised the fluoride level four to six times higher than topical and 50-70 times higher than control teeth. In the seventh etch, iontophoresis raised the fluoride level about 5 times higher than topical and 28-40 times higher than control teeth. In other words, the electrical current forces more fluoride into the teeth and to a greater depth than topical application. We believe this increase of fluoride may be enough to precipitate CaF_2 crystals which physically block the tubules and which are trapped deeply in the tubules. This trapping could result in more perfect mineralization because F^- ion absorbed into the tubular fluid could exchange for hydroxyl radicals in hydroxyapatite to form fluorapatite. On the other hand topical application may only form the CaF_2 at or near the surface which can then be readily reabsorbed into the saliva diminishing the chance of reaction with tooth mineral.

This review and discussion clearly indicate that the mechanism of fluoride desensitization is not well understood. A better understanding may be obtained when greater knowledge about the mechanisms of dentin sensation is received and also through study of effects of fluoride reactions in the dentinal tubules.

Chapter 4

Rationale for Treating Oral Lesions

Oral lesions of three types have been found to be successfully treated by iontophoresis in the author's experience:

1. Canker sores or aphthous lesions, including periadenitis mucosa necrotica recurrens (PMNR);
2. Lichen planus, and
3. Cold sores or herpes simplex orolabialis.

Aphthous Lesions (canker sores)

According to Leyden (Conn's Cur. Ther., 1975) the treatments for oral aphthous ulcers are:

1. Steroid in an adherent vehicle (Kenalog in Orabase[R]) four times daily;
2. Tetracycline compresses, four times daily;
3. Silver nitrate to cauterize the lesion, and
4. Lidocaine viscous four times daily.

Silver nitrate and other caustic agents may give temporary relief by action on nerve endings and protecting the surface, but healing time is not decreased. Lidocaine or other local anesthetics give only temporary relief.
Graykowski and Holroyd[35] reviewed the treatment of aphthous ulcers concluding that an oral rinse of tetracycline suspension or topical corticosteroids are the most effective methods of treatment. For both types of drugs, the treatment was most effective when started very early in the course of the disease. According to Graykowski, persistent oral ulceration with continuous lesions and constant discomfort may require systemic therapy with steroids. However, he warned of the dangers of systemic steroids in causing adrenocortical suppression. Since aphthae may often result in constant discomfort, the dentist needs an effective treatment which will avoid the danger of systemic toxicity. We have been reluctant to use systemic steroids because of this danger.
Since iontophoresis allows local treatment with powerful drugs without any danger of systemic adverse effects, the iontophoresis of steroids directly into aphthous lesions was studied. The results were dramatic. A single treatment with the charged steroid, methylprednisolone sodium succinate (Solu-Medrol[R]) was effective in giving immediate relief, elimination of inflammation and rapid healing.
A typical example of the immediate changes and rapid healing obtained after steroid iontophoresis is demonstrated in Figures 9a, b and c. Figure 9a shows an aphthous lesion in the corner of the mouth before treatment. The patient was a healthy 35-year-old female who had aphthae recurring constantly so that she was rarely without a lesion. Her usual heal-

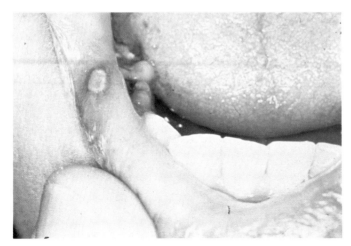

Figs. 9a, 9b and 9c Aphthous lesion treated by iontophoresis.

Fig. 9a Before iontophoresis.

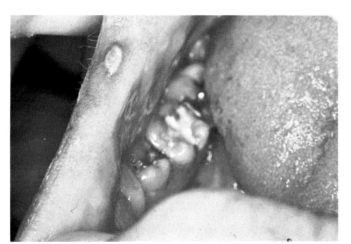

Fig. 9b After iontophoresis (immediate).

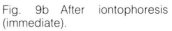
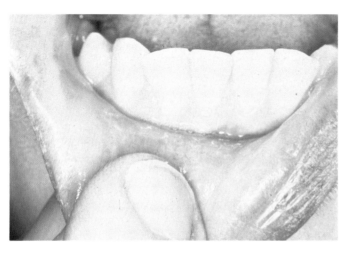

Fig. 9c After iontophoresis (3 days).

ing time was 14-21 days. The lesion on the corner of the mouth (Fig. 9a) had been present for 3 days and was progressively getting worse; because of the movement of the mouth; this seemed to irritate the lesion and cause a great amount of discomfort. Solu-Medrol[R] iontophoresis was applied at the cathode at 0.4 mA for 5 minutes. Immediately after removing the electrode (Fig. 9b), there was a numb feeling but the numbness disappeared in 2-5 minutes and the discomfort was relieved. In this case, the lips were much more mobile and three days later the area was completely healed (Fig. 9c).

Most adrenocorticosteroids are uncharged, but Solu-Medrol[R] was designed for intravenous use and water solubility by chemical synthesis which converts the steroid base into salt form. Solu-Medrol[R] is negatively charged and is applied over the lesion using the negative electrode to assure a high concentration of drug in the lesion. Very rarely, the patient requires a second treatment one or two days later. In such cases, it was often found that local trauma from lip or cheek biting, excessive plaque or poor restorations was a contributing factor. The dentist should check for such perpetuating factors in all cases before performing any recommended therapy.

In the early stages of development of the Solu-Medrol[R] iontophoresis, the author found some difficulty in treating lesions near the tongue, or in highly vascular areas. It was assumed that the poor results were due to a rapid removal of the steroid by the profuse vascularity of the area. A technique was therefore developed to, first, vasoconstrict the area and then, apply the steroid. Epinephrine hydrochloride iontophoresis is used for vasoconstriction; two steps are required since epinephrine is positively charged, while Solu-Medrol[R] is negatively charged. Adrenaline HCL[R] diluted to about 1/25,000 is

first iontophoresed to the lesion for two minutes under the positive electrode, then the steroid is iontophoresed for 4 minutes under the negative electrode. Figures 10a, b and c demonstrate results obtained by the two-step method. Figure 10a shows an aphthous lesion in a 24-year-old healthy female who was plagued with lesions constantly. Her orthodontic bands seemed to irritate the lips and many lesions frequently occurred, mainly in the lower lip, but sometimes in other areas. Figure 10b shows the lesion immediately after epinephrine iontophoresis at 0.3 mA for 3 min. The vasoconstriction obtained is obvious. Figure 10c shows the lesion immediately after Solu-Medrol[R] iontophoresis. In this case, there was a changed appearance of the lesion, the typical numbness for a few minutes, loss of discomfort and rapid healing in 4 days.

Recently, we have found that patients with large, uncomfortable lesions were made more comfortable during the procedure by applying local anesthetics. We start by applying lidocaine ointment, 5%. The ointment is removed and 2% lidocaine with 1/50,000 epinephrine is iontophoresed under the positive electrode. This provides both vasoconstriction and deep topical anesthesia. Both of these drugs are positive, ions and can be introduced at the same time. The standard solution from a dental cartridge appears to be effective for this procedure. Then the Solu-Medrol[R] iontophoresis is performed under the negative electrode.

The author has made no attempt to systematically evaluate tetracycline therapy for aphthous ulceration.

In conclusion, the Solu-Medrol[R] iontophoresis appears to give a very beneficial effect in aphthous ulceration. Discomfort is relieved and healing time greatly reduced. Details of all the methods for treating aphthae are presented in Chapter 15.

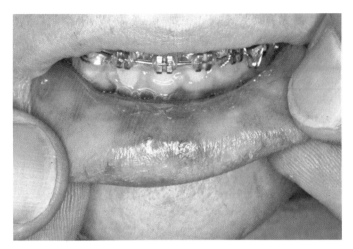

Figs. 10a, 10b and 10c Two step method of aphthous ulcer treatment.

Fig. 10a   Before iontophoresis.

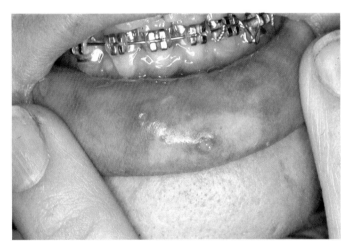

Fig. 10b After epinephrine iontophoresis.

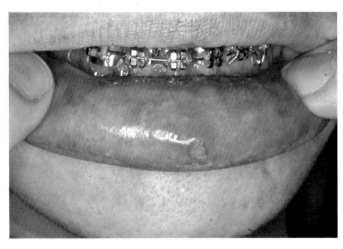

Fig. 10c After Solu-Medrol® iontophoresis.

Lichen Planus

There appears to be no effective treatment currently available for lichen planus. Leyden[62] recommends administration of steroids topically, systemically or by intralesional injection.

Topical steroid treatment appears difficult because of problems of penetration and keeping the drug on the lesion. Since the lesions may be quite large, intralesional injection requires multiple needle placement which does not result in even drug distribution. Also a great deal of drug may be used resulting in local atrophy and possible systemic steroid effect. Although Conn indicates that systemic therapy may be necessary, the dangers of systemic therapy may outweigh the benefits received. Therefore, we have tried the Solu-Medrol[R] iontophoresis and found it to be extremely effective in converting the erosive, inflammatory type of lichen planus to the less bothersome fibrous pattern. The number of cases we have done is small but the results appear promising. A course of three treatments is used and repeated 1-3 times yearly if needed.

Herpes Orolabialis (cold sores, herpes simplex infection)

There is currently no accepted treatment for Herpesvirus (HSV-1) lesions of the orofacial region. Several antiviral compounds are available. Iododeoxyuridine (IDU, idoxuridine) is an antiviral compound (Kaufman[55] which has been shown to be effective, by topical application, in eye infections caused by HSV-1. Stoxil[R], Dendrid[R] and Herplex[R] are preparations of IDU which have been on the market for about 15 years and used extensively for HSV-1 infections of the eye, in the form of 0.1% ophthalmic solution. Recently, IDU ointment (0.5%) has been marketed for the same purpose. Also, Vira-A[R] (Ara-A) has been introduced for HSV-1 eye infection.[44] Unfortunately, these preparations have not been shown to be effective in treatment of cutaneous infections.[72] The problem seems to be lack of penetration because these drugs are powerful antiviral compounds when used *in vitro*.[77]

Gangarosa, Park and Hill[19] studied penetration of IDU into mouse skin and found that cathodal iontophoresis greatly assisted the penetration compared to topical application. While the area of skin treated had a high concentration of IDU, the systemic dose was very small; the amount appearing in blood or in liver was the same as for topical application (Gangarosa, unpublished observations). Although IDU may be a dangerous drug when used systemically in large doses, topical use is considered safe; iontophoretic application gives an additional safety factor because one application usually gives a dramatic reduction of the lesion followed by rapid healing. Occasionally the treatment is repeated one time, but we have never found it necessary to use a third treatment.

The safety of iontophoretic application of Stoxil[R] is indicated by the following calculations. The topical dose in the eye is 2 drops (0.1cc) every hour during waking hours and 2 drops every 2 hours at night (assume 16 waking hours and 8 hours of sleep with therapy necessary for 4 days at full dosage and 4 days at a reduced dosage [$1/2$]).

16 doses   = 1.6 cc
× 0.1 cc/dose
4 doses   = 0.4 cc
× 0.1 cc/dose
         2.0 cc daily
         ×4   days
         8.0 cc
         4.0 cc (4 days ½ dosage)
         12.0 cc

Dose delivered by iontophoresis = 0.03 cc (0.3 cc × 10% of drug absorbed; calculated from unpublished experimental data of Gangarosa and Park)

Safety factor $= \dfrac{12}{0.03} = 400$

Thus, iontophoresis is 400 times safer than topical eye treatment. According to the manufacturer (PDR, 1978) . . . "the minimum systemic dose that will produce toxic effects is many times greater than the quantity in a commercial bottle (15 mg). . ."

The author studied herpes labialis treatment by iontophoresis of Stoxil[R],[28] and concluded that it is extremely effective with reduction of healing time to 3-4 days (normal 9-10 days). There was immediate loss of discomfort and acceleration of all subsequent stages of the lesions, including coalescence of vesicles, rapid oozing, appearance of a small scab, lack of spread of lesions and rapid healing. From the toxicological considerations (see above) the author concludes that the technique is ultrasafe with no possibility of systemic reactions. Nevertheless, there are three contraindications to the use of Stoxil[R] iontophoresis: 1) allergy to the drug (the author has not found any patient who reports allergy): 2) pregnancy, especially first trimester (one report,[46] claimed that IDU is teratogenic); and 3) where there is little benefit to be obtained (the greater the benefit, the greater the benefit/risk ratio).

1. Indications (where the patient will benefit) from Stoxil[R] iontophoresis include:
   a. History of spread of the lesions to other parts of the body, especially the eye.
   b. To prevent spread of infections in persons who are liable to have a disastrous generalized herpes infection such as, (1) small infants (treat the mother or nursery workers) or (2) immune compromised person (treat family or hospital personnel).
   c. Massive recurrent attack involving one-fourth or more of the lips and generally interfering with alimentation, speech and appearance.
   d. Interference with one's profession, such as a speaker or a wind-instrument player.
   e. An immune-compromised patient where the virus could spread to other organs.
   f. Any primary attack.

2. Safety Factors:
   a. Amount of drug used in iontophoretic treatment is extremely minute.
   b. The drug is highly localized to the lip.
   c. The effectiveness of iontophoresis (high concentration of drug at the active site) makes induction of viral resistance unlikely.
   d. An effective drug treatment should reduce the possibility of inactivated virus inducing cancer, since less virus would be produced following treatment.

3. Risks:
   a. There is a remote, *theoretical* possibility that the drug will induce mutations of human cells which may lead to cancer. This possibility seems to be outweighed by the more likely (but also theoretical) possibility that the virus will induce cancer.

b. Induction of viral drug resistance. Viral resistance should occur less frequently if a high dose of drug is delivered to the active site. Since iontophoresis favors penetration into the skin,[19] there should be less chance for induction of viral resistance when iontophoresis is used, compared to topical administration.

Our initial preliminary experiments with IDU iontophoresis were reported at the International Association for Dental Research.[18,28] In each of six patients, one lesion was allowed to follow its natural course; the mean time to complete healing was 8.8 days. One or more lesions in each patient was treated by IDU iontophoresis. Mean healing time was reduced about 63% to 3.4 days. There was immediate relief of discomfort and accelerated healing in all treated cases. These results were so promising that an early report in the literature[28] seemed appropriate, even though the trials were not blinded.

Some typical results obtained by IDU iontophoresis of herpes simplex lesions are described in several case reports.

Case 1 - Patient GL

GL was referred by an allergist for treatment of frequent chronic attacks of RHL. This 28-year-old female was in good health except for numerous allergies and a major complaint of recurrent herpes labialis. The history of these lesions was typical with prodromal signs, appearance of papular stage and vesicles early in the lesion (1-2 days), spreading of lesions to involve the entire lip and sometimes both lips, and a 10-12 day healing time. When one lesion healed another would appear; thus, she was treated on five occasions between April 25 and July 17, 1975. On each occasion prodromal lesions were treated with IDU iontophoresis. Improvement was noticed immediately after each treatment. In one trial, several small vesicles were present; they coalesced immediately after treatment to resemble a later stage of the lesion. Vesicle coalescence is demonstrated in Figures 11a and b. Figure 11a shows a typical lesion before therapy and Figure 11b shows the lesion immediately after therapy. In addition, discomfort was alleviated and the overall lesion did not enlarge. Within 1-2 days, the lesion oozed and a slight scab occurred in 2-3 days when swelling disappeared. Healing was essentially complete in five days.

The untreated lesion in this patient healed in 14 days with spread of lesions to contiguous areas of the lip, much oozing, some tissue necrosis and a large scab.

Case 2 - Patient LPG

The author was the patient, thus, allowing specific temporal observation of the clinical response. He was a healthy 45-year-old male who had had frequent attacks of herpes simplex over a period of 30 years. Healing usually required 7-10 days with spread of lesions and a great amount of discomfort and scabbing in the later stages. The untreated lesion in this patient healed in 7 days. The treated lesion was only 4 hours old and considered prodromal with no vesicles evident. Immediately after treatment vesicles appeared. The burning and itching sensation diminished following treatment, and swelling was reduced. After two hours, the swelling seemed to return (increasing slightly); six hours later, swelling was reduced again. The area of the lesion was slightly sensitive, although not uncomfortable, for 30 hours after treatment. After about 36 hours sensitivity of the lesion had disappeared. Forty hours after treatment, a small amount

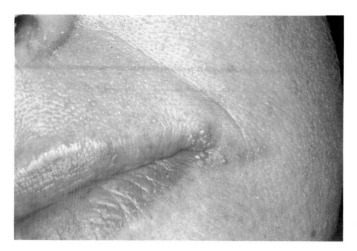

Figs. 11a and 11b Idoxuridine iontophoresis in subject GL.

Fig. 11a Immediately before iontophoresis.

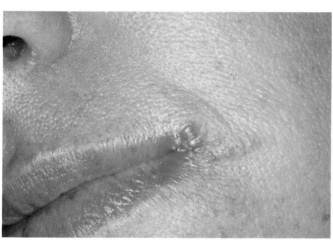

Fig. 11b Several minutes after iontophoresis. (Notice the coalescence of vesicles at the angle of the lips.)

of fluid and scab were removed from the lesion and healing appeared almost complete. Figures 12a and b show this lesion before treatment (Fig. 12a) and 40 hours later (Fig. 12b) demonstrating the accelerated healing of the lesion, which occurs following IDU iontophoresis.

Case 3 - Patient DG

This case was not described in the publication[28] but illustrates the occasional need

for a second treatment. Subject DG was a 48-year-old healthy female with a history of multiple recurrent attacks of herpes labialis. The lesion was on the upper left lip near the nose and was 2 cm diameter, indurated, swollen and in the papular stage. Figure 13a shows the lesion before IDU iontophoresis. The treatment was applied for 10 min; relief of discomfort and appearance of vesicles may be noted in Figure 13b immediately after treatment. Forty-eight hours later the lesion had not completely healed and some induration was

Figs. 12a and 12b Idoxuridine iontophoresis on subject LPG.

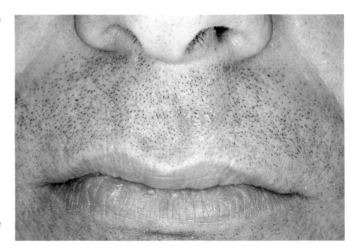

Fig. 12a Immediately before iontophoresis.

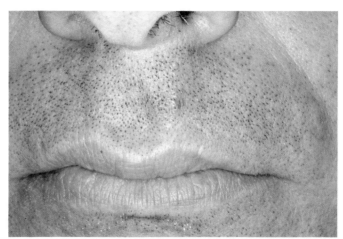

Fig. 12b Two days after iontophoresis. (The lesion is arrested and is almost healed.)

still present (Fig. 13c). It was felt that the patient would benefit from a second treatment because the lesion was still late and induration had returned. The result after the second treatment is shown in Figure 13d. The lesion wept profusely, crusted and was almost completely healed in 2 more days. The scab formed shortly after and fell off after 5 days.

In conclusion, the IDU (Stoxil^R) iontophoresis appears effective for treatment of herpes orolabialis, while the risk of any side effects appears almost nonexistent.

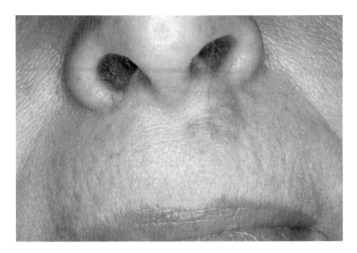

Figs. 13a, 13b, 13c and 13d Idoxuridine iontophoresis in subject DG.

Fig. 13a Immediately before iontophoresis.

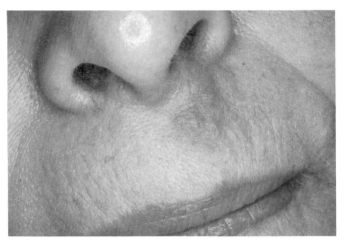

Fig. 13b Immediately after iontophoresis. Notice the lesion is not as diffuse and is less inflamed.

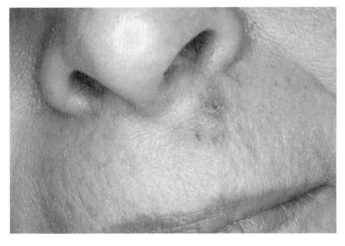

Fig. 13c Two days later. Although improved there was still some induration, therefore a second IDU treatment was given.

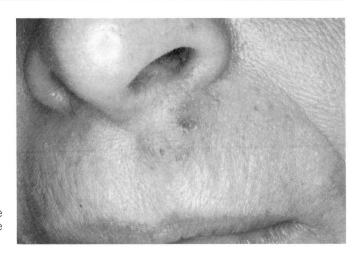

Fig. 13d Immediately after the second treatment. Complete healing occurred in 3 days.

Chapter 5

Rationale for Local Anesthesia of Oral Mucosa

In 1974, the author[16] reported that iontophoresis of 2% lidocaine with 1/25,000 epinephrine was effective for producing deep surface anesthesia of the oral mucosa for the extraction of loose deciduous teeth. The procedures used were effective for removing twelve deciduous teeth, in 3 patients, over a period of three years. The methods used in performing the trials are shown in Figures 14a, b, c and d and 15. The oral electrode was formed as described in Figures 14a, b and c. This saddle-shaped electrode was fitted over the mucosa around the loose deciduous tooth (Fig. 15) with local anesthetic solution (2% lidocaine and 1/25,000 epinephrine) saturating the cotton (Fig. 14c). A positive charge was applied by connecting the oral electrode to the anode. The skin (return) electrode (Fig. 14d) is similar to electrodes used for performing cystic fibrosis analysis. It was found that 1 mA of current for 5-10 minutes produced adequate anesthesia for forceps removal of the teeth without any pain. Following iontophoresis, maximum anesthesia was achieved in 2-3 minutes. If a fairly long root was present, a small amount of 2% lidocaine with 1/50,000 epinephrine was injected into the anesthetized mucosa on the side of the long root. When anesthesia was complete, a normal extraction was performed.

Table 4 describes the results of this study. For extraction in trials 1 through 10, iontophoresis of the local anesthetic was performed for 10 minutes. Current was applied in trials 11 and 12 for only five minutes, whereas for trial 13 the current was applied for 15 minutes. Two to three minutes after the removal of electrodes, the teeth were luxated by finger pressure to determine any change in sensation. The patients indicated that this procedure was without discomfort as compared to that experienced before application of iontophoresis, although they still felt pressure. A straight elevator and forceps were then used to complete the extraction. Twelve of the 13 teeth were extracted satisfactorily, and the patient experienced no pain or discomfort. One patient experienced a slight degree of unpleasantness during extraction in trial 7. The mouth electrode was still under development at that time; adaption of the electrode to tissue was not considered adequate.

In trial 2, a rather long remaining root on X-ray was noted; it was decided to infiltrate local anesthetic by injection into the site previously anesthetized by iontophoresis in order to obtain deeper anesthesia around the bony attachment. The patient felt no discomfort from needle insertion on either the labial or the palatal aspect. Because of a lack of mobility, current was applied in trial 13, for 15 minutes. A completely satisfactory anesthesia for more than an hour was obtained.

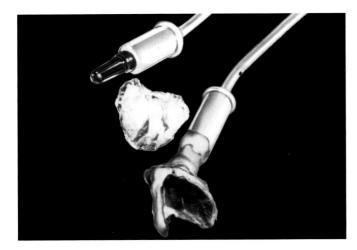

Figs. 14a, 14b, 14c and 14d Electrodes for deciduous tooth extraction.

Fig. 14a Electrode plug that fits into iontophoresis apparatus; aluminum foil adapted, covered with cotton, that fits into mouth electrode; saddle-shaped electrode that holds drug against tissue to be anesthetized.

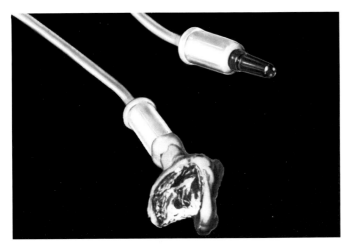

Fig. 14b Aluminum foil adapted to mouth electrode.

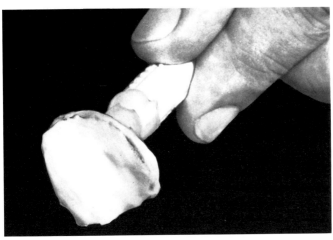

Fig. 14c Mouth electrode completely assembled.

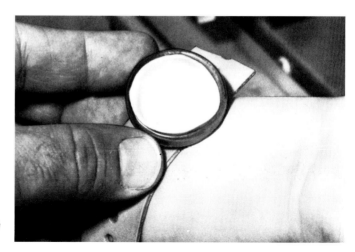

Fig. 14d Indifferent electrode applied to skin over wrist.

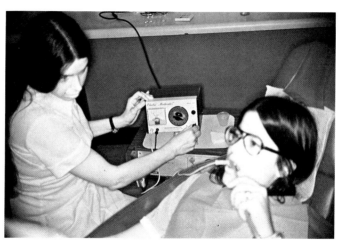

Fig. 15 Iontophoresor (AC rectifier) completely connected for use. Note positive electrode (white) attached at area of local anesthesia application. Indifferent electrode (black) is attached to arm (attachment not shown in Fig. 15, see Fig. 6).

Summary

Using only iontophoresis for anesthesia of the periodontal mucosa, 12 deciduous anterior teeth were extracted. The time of iontophoresis varied from 5 to 15 minutes. One other tooth was extracted after the use of iontophoresis and the painless injection of local anesthetic into the anesthetized mucosa. Local anesthesia by injection would have been advisable for extraction of all 13 teeth, if iontophoresis had not been used. Twelve of the 13 extractions were considered successful in that the patients felt no discomfort. Discomfort in one patient was attributed to technical difficulties during development of the mouth electrode.

We now recommend this technique for obtaining anesthesia before extraction of all loose deciduous teeth. Because of the sound theoretical basis for recommending this technique, a large scale trial was not done. There is adequate precedence for use of iontophoresis for surface anesthesia. Harris[40] outlined the technique for

Table 4 Deciduous Teeth Extracted by Iontophoresis

Patient	Age	Trial number	Tooth	Mobility* (mm)	Root length (cm)	Method of anesthesia[†]	Current duration (min)
Boy	12	1	Maxillary right canine	2	0.4	E	10
	13	2	Maxillary left canine	0	1.3	E & injection	10
Girl	7	3	Mandibular left central incisor	3	0.3	E	10
	8	4	Mandibular right lateral incisor	2	0.5	E	10
	8	5	Maxillary right central incisor	3	0.4	E	10
	8	6	Maxillary left central incisor	3	0.4	E	10
Girl	6	7	Mandibular right central incisor	3	0.4	E	10
	6	8	Mandibular left central incisor	4	0.2	E	10
	7	9	Mandibular left lateral incisor	2	0.3	E	10
	7	10	Mandibular right lateral incisor	3	0.3	E	10
	7	11	Maxillary right central incisor	2	0.4	E	5
	7	12	Maxillary left central incisor	2	0.4	E	5
	8	13	Maxillary right lateral incisor	1	0.3[‡]	E	15

*Labial-lingual movement of incisal edge for discomfort end point
[†]E, electrical medication (iontophoresis).
[‡]This root was not completely resorbed lingually; this accounts for the lack of mobility.

introducing local anesthetics and epinephrine hydrochloride at the same time, under the anode. Comeau et al.[11] studied a similar use of iontophoresis for anesthesia of the ear drum. Echols et al.[12] further studied the Comeau technique and the Editor of *Eye, Ear, Nose & Throat*[45] considered the use of iontophoretic local anesthesia as a major advancement. The author[26] reported on studies defining the iontophoretic solution for skin anesthesia. Controlled experiments showed that epinephrine hydrochloride was a necessary component of the solution, but the concentration used by the author for oral mucosa or skin anesthesia was much less (1/12,500-1/50,000), than was used by Comeau group (1/2,000) or by Echols.

Further it was observed that none of the following were effective in producing skin anesthesia; saline solution with current, epinephrine solution alone or with current, lidocaine solution alone or with current, or lidocaine and epinephrine solution without current. There seemed to be no advantage in increasing lidocaine concentration from 2% to 4%. While on a theoretical basis the presence of other salts in the anesthetic solution would compete for current (supposedly reducing effectiveness) there was no discernible difference between the dental local anesthetic from cartridge (2% lidocaine with 1/50,000 epinephrine, containing 0.10 M solution chloride), and a solution with similar lidocaine-epinephrine concentrations without the added salt. The latter observation indicates that the iontophoresis technique can be used with Xylocaine[R], green dental anesthetic cartridge. Nevertheless, on a theoretical basis, an ideal solution for oral mucosal anesthesia would be 4% lidocaine hydrochloride (one - 5 ml ampule for medical use) mixed with 0.5 ml of 1/1000 epinephrine hydrochloride (1 ml ampule for medical use). This solution must be mixed fresh daily. Many deciduous tooth extractions have been completed by the author and his students using modifications of the methods described in his original paper.[16] The new methodology will be thoroughly detailed in Chapter 14.

The author has also found that iontophoretic application of lidocaine hydrochloride with epinephrine hydrochloride is effective for preinjection topical anesthesia. Current is applied at 1 mA for 3-5 minutes. This procedure is especially effective prior to palatal injections. If the dental assistant prepares the injection sites by iontophoresis, there would be an actual saving of time by the dentist.

The iontophoretic local anesthesia is also suitable for biopsy. Use of ionto-phoretic local anesthesia is under study for lancing of abscesses.

A child's first encounter with a dentist is usually critical; modern pedodontics teaches us to see the child early (before any dental problems have developed), in order to train the child as a cooperative patient. Unfortunately, many parents wait until the child needs to have a tooth extracted before dragging the reluctant patient to the dentist. It would be advantageous to extract the loose deciduous tooth without the prospect of an injection at the first appointment, but all of our previous methods to avoid the needle have failed. Now the use of iontophoresis eliminates the need for the needle insertion at the child's first appointment.

Further, a profound topical anesthesia can be obtained before needle insertion using iontophoresis of lidocaine and epinephrine. There are many dental patients who fear the dental appointment, because of the discomfort of needle insertion. Our present emphasis, in reducing patient anxiety, is in using intravenous drugs; yet, if the patient fears a needle, injecting into a vein does not seem to be a satisfactory substitute, and, if difficulty is encountered, the procedure of finding a vein may be traumatic.

For the anxious patient, iontophoresis could help to eliminate the fear of needle insertion, as well as the need for systemic drug therapy for anxiety control. Preinjection topical anesthesia by iontophoresis is recommended before injection into sensitive areas, such as the palate.

It is also possible, using palatal stints or saddle-shaped electrodes which fit over the gingiva, to completely eliminate injections for palatal anesthesia or for gingival curettage. The procedures for use of trays and stints will be described in Chapter 14.

Chapter 6

Conclusions and Perspectives

The subject of iontophoresis must be viewed in terms of methods of drug administration. The major methods of administration are systemic (or parenteral) and topical (or local). Parenteral administration is favored when the disease affects the entire body, or when the effect desired is in a tissue which is not accessible from the surface. Since parenteral administration involves the risk of adverse side effects, topical administration is preferred when the condition to be treated is accessible from the body surface. In topical administration, side effects are limited to the tissue under treatment, provided the drug is not absorbed systemically or is absorbed very slowly.

It is apparent that there is a dilemma in topical therapy. If the drug is well absorbed, then the dangers of topical application are the same as for systemic application. This has been noted for potent, well-absorbed drugs such as tetracaine[4] or epinephrine;[3] for such agents, the topical dose is the same as the systemic therapeutic dose. On the other hand, if the drug is absorbed very slowly, it may not reach a high enough concentration in the surface tissue.

The advantages of iontophoresis are now very apparent. When a surface of the body requires drug therapy, iontophoretic administration assures penetration of the drug and a high concentration in the surface under treatment, while the total dose delivered to the entire body, is infinitesimally low. In his treatise, Leduc[57] questioned the exposure of the entire body to a risk of adverse drug effects, if one desires the drug effect in only a localized area.

In dentistry, we deal almost entirely with surface tissues. Further, the dentist is and should be reluctant to treat the entire body, when he desires an effect in the tooth or in the oral mucosa. Naturally, if the problem is systemic, the dentist should attempt systemic therapy, but local therapy may still be advisable in the beginning in order to rule out local factors. Thus, local therapy is most important to dental practice.

Iontophoresis would be helpful to dentists in many situations where it is desired to apply drugs in the oral cavity with assurance of drug penetration. Iontophoresis is essential for treating hypersensitive dentin in the dental office. The fluoride iontophoresis seems to be the only truly effective treatment for dentin exposure. All other topical and home care treatments appear to be only slightly more effective or equal to placebo treatments.

The fluoride iontophoresis is biologically safe and meets the criteria of an ideal tooth desensitizer. Dentin desensitization is required for any type of dentin exposure including cervical erosion, cervical abrasion, occlusal wear, exposure after periodontal surgery, exposure during restorative treatment, hypoplastic enamel and open dentino-cemental junction.

The patient that has exposed dentin may develop extreme sensitivity which causes constant discomfort (pain) from temperature changes, air flow in the oral cavity or imbibing acrid foods and liquids. This discomfort may be with the patient at all times. The dentist will be a better practitioner if he can effectively treat hypersensitive exposed dentin which is either present when the patient is first seen or which develops during the course of treatment.

The author concludes that the fluoride iontophoresis is a necessary component of dental practice. Every dentist should have the iontophoresis equipment available either in his own office or by referral. All dental schools should teach the fluoride iontophoresis so that the dentist of tomorrow will be sufficiently acquainted with the technique that he will offer this service as part of his practice. Dental schools and the dental profession should also take on the responsibility of educating practitioners in iontophoresis.

Iontophoresis is also useful in obtaining a better mucosal anesthesia for use as a preinjection topical or for extraction of loose deciduous teeth without the necessity of an injection. The esteem of dental patients for the dentist is increased when he takes all possible care in his injection technique. Any method of eliminating dental pain from needle injections will be a great aid to dental practice by eliminating patient anxiety. Iontophoresis of local anesthetics and epinephrine will be useful in dental practice as an aid to pain and anxiety control.

The present method of topically applying local anesthetics in ointments is rather ineffective; it provides only a slight and superficial numbness. Many dentists have disbanded use of topicals because of their ineffectiveness. The author regards this trend as detrimental to good patient care and pain-anxiety control. The author believes that the dental profession should foster any method of improving topical anesthesia. Iontophoresis will assure penetration of local anesthetics and epinephrine, providing the dentists with a truly effective preinjection topical. This will be useful because most dental patients perceive injections as one of the most threatening factors in their dental care.[64]

The treatment of oral lesions is a third major use of iontophoresis in dental practice. Currently, the treatment of aphthous lesions by dentists involves the use of a number of remedies, many of which are old fashioned and only as effective as placebos. Some of these remedies contain caustic substances and are of no benefit in reducing healing time. Although steroids in adherent ointments appear to be of some value, most areas of the oral cavity are not well-adapted to allow adherence. A more positive way to assure penetration of anti-inflammatory steroids is through iontophoresis. Solu-Medrol[R] is a charged, anti-inflammatory steroid which can be introduced into oral lesions which have no known etiology. The author concludes that the Solu-Medrol[R] iontophoresis is effective for aphthous ulcer (canker sore) and lichen planus treatment. Iontophoresis will be useful in dental practice for treating such nonspecific inflammatory lesions.

The dentist has no specific therapy for viral lesions of the lip. Cold sores (herpes orolabialis) are caused by herpes simplex virus (HSV). Some patients have HSV lesions only occasionally and the lesions often heal uneventfully. This type of lesion should *not* be treated. However, many patients have numerous lesions that heal slowly. The lesions may be painful and may interfere with the patient's daily activities. Examples of patients who should benefit from an effective antiviral treatment include: a mother with a small infant, a nurse who works with infants or immune-compromised patients, a patient with a history of spread of the infection to the eye, a patient with a festering infection which is not healing, a patient with a primary attack, and a patient who requires use of mouth in his livelihood (wind musician, speaker, etc.).

The author has found that the idoxuridine (Stoxil[R]) iontophoresis is useful for the patient who will obtain a definite benefit from the treatment. Idoxuridine is an antiviral drug which is acceptable for human use for treatment of HSV infections of the eye. The idoxuridine iontophoresis for herpes labialis is much safer even than topical administration in the eye. The author concludes that iontophoresis of idoxuridine is a useful aid in dental practice for treating selected patients who will receive a definite benefit from the treatment.

If the dentist adopts the technique of iontophoresis, he will be able to administer drugs by this method for other conditions. The author believes that most drugs can be administered more effectively and more safely by iontophoresis than by topical or systemic administration. The technique may be useful: for aiding fluoride penetration of enamel during topical therapy; for administration of epinephrine and other drugs directly into the gingiva; for more effective pain control of hypersensitive teeth during endodontics allowing dentin and pulp tissue removal; for local anesthesia of abscesses before lancing; for tetracycline or antibiotic treatment of infections; for anti-inflammatory steroid treatment of pulpal tissue, either directly or through dentin. The dentist may also think of other conditions he would like to treat, where drugs are available, and apply the principles of iontophoresis to the problem.

The principles of iontophoresis are:

1. Condition to be treated is at or accessible from a body surface,
2. Drug to be used is charged;
3. Charged drug is applied at appropriate electrode of the same charge;
4. Return electrode of the same or larger area is applied to another site on the body;
5. Indifferent electrolyte is used to saturate the return electrode;
6. Metal or highly conductive electrode material must not contact the body;
7. Adjacent areas which may conduct current, such as gingiva or metallic restorations must be insulated;
8. A safe amount of current (below patient's threshold of sensation) is applied for an appropriate length of time; and
9. Safety rules (maximum current, current-duration, etc.) are observed.

In Section II of this monograph, we will consider some important scientific principles related to use of iontophoresis and diagnosis of the conditions to be treated.

Section II

Scientific Principles of Iontophoretic Treatment

Chapter 7

Science and Logic Applied to Iontophoresis

Iontophoresis has had a long history in health care for delivery of drugs to the body. The technique of drug delivery by electrical current was first suggested as the physical laws of electricity were being described, e.g., medication by ions was recommended by Faraday, Volta, and others. (For a complete review of the history of iontophoresis, see Chapter 2). One may logically ask, "If iontophoresis has been available for so many years, why hasn't it become a popular method of therapy?" The answer to this question has many facets. Certainly, from time to time, researchers have studied the technique of iontophoresis and shown some enthusiasm by publishing one or more papers. Yet, it appears that, until recently, no group of researchers has made a concerted effort to define the scientific basis for iontophoresis, its usefulness and its limitations. The monograph of Abramowitsch and Neoussikine[2] is illustrative of the state of the art at that time. They mentioned numerous uses for iontophoresis in medical practice, but they presented no data; claims for various successes were totally unsupported. Furthermore, most of the claims were rather extravagant, e.g., claims for therapy of schizophrenia or of deep muscle scars. O'Malley and Oester[73] ushered in the scientific era of iontophoresis. They proved that the drug is concentrated only in tissue touching the electrode surface and does not follow the complete pathway of the current. This finding sets the limits for iontophoresis; the technique is only useful for treatment of surface tissues. It is theoretically possible to use iontophoresis for systemic therapy, since the drug which localizes in the tissue is absorbed into the blood stream, but it is not possible to direct the drug at a specified organ, below the surface of the body unless contact is made between electrode and tissue to be treated.

Harris[40] outlined a number of rational uses for iontophoresis in medicine, but some of the uses he described were beyond the limits of the technique. Gibson and Cooke[31] gave iontophoresis research a great impetus by their recommendation of pilocarpine nitrate iontophoresis for cystic fibrosis diagnosis. As a result, iontophoresis is being used, many times daily, on infants and small children, in almost every major medical center in the U.S.A.

A second major use for iontophoresis has developed out of the work of J. Vernon and his colleagues at the University of Oregon (1973). They showed that lidocaine-epinephrine iontophoresis is safe and effective for local anesthesia of the ear drum prior to myringotomy. This significant advancement, which only requires a few minutes, is important because it replaces general anesthesia for this painful operation. Sisler[90] adopted the same technique for minor surgery of the cornea. The author,[16] working independently, reported anesthesia of the oral mucosa by lidocaine-epinephrine iontophoresis at about the same time as the Vernon report. Recently, S. Jacobsen and co-workers,[47] at the University of Utah, reported excellent anesthesia of skin using lidocaine iontophoresis.

About 1964, the author first realized the possibilities of iontophoresis. This technique, if properly applied, appeared to be a pharmacologist's dream, i.e., a drug can be placed exactly at the site where it is most needed, without affecting other organs of the body, thereby eliminating systemic side effects. There appeared to be broad possibilities for therapeutic applications, because of the availability of a great number of potent, modern drugs. In the next few years, the author experimented with local anesthesia of the skin, following the methods outlined by Harris (1959). As a result, the oral mucosal anesthesia by iontophoresis for extraction of loose deciduous teeth was reported.[16] This topic was interesting to the author, not only to eliminate needle injection at a child's first appointment, but also because, during his practice of dentistry, many patients had indicated a fear of needle injection, which was a cause of anxiety. How wonderful it would be to have a technique which would make the practice of pain control so much more effective, thereby eliminating patient fear and anxiety! Now it is available! No patient has to suffer from pain of a palatal injection henceforth, if the dentist will adopt the technique of topical anesthesia by iontophoresis.

Having met with this success, the author turned his attention, in 1971, to other problems of dental practice which could be solved by iontophoretic medication. It soon became apparent that dental therapy involves, to a large extent, surfaces of the oral cavity. Since iontophoresis is mainly suitable for treating tissues at body surfaces, it follows that there are many applications of iontophoresis in dental practice. The author was particularly interested in developing therapies for conditions which are not amenable to usual dental therapy. The dentist tends to neglect hypersensitive teeth, aphthous ulcers, and herpes labialis because good treatments are not available. Yet patients with these problems are in pain and discomfort and should not be neglected. Very often, such patients become sources of anxiety to the dentist because he realizes their need for pain relief but he is unable to do anything about it.

The author therefore adopted the principles of iontophoresis described below as guidelines for the application of drugs in resolving some difficult dental problems.

Selection of the Drug of Choice

The drug of choice may be an agent currently used by topical application or a well-accepted drug for similar condition in another part of the body.

The drug of choice for hypersensitive teeth appeared to be fluoride ion because of moderate success reported by topical application. It could be surmised that the fluoride ion would be more effective in desensitizing hypersensitive dentin if a greater rate of penetration could be obtained. Indeed, a number of reports (see Chapter 3) indicated that fluoride iontophoresis was probably more effective than topical application. The controlled, clinical study of Murphy[71] reported 1% sodium fluoride iontophoresis to be superior to topical application of 33 $\frac{1}{3}$% sodium fluoride paste. Nevertheless, there appeared to be many problems which would not allow general acceptance of iontophoresis into dental practice (see next page). The author used scientific principles to develop a

Drug of Choice	Charge	Condition
fluoride ion	−	hypersensitive dentin
methyl prednisolone succinate (sodium salt)	−	inflammation
idoxuridine	−	herpes labialis
lidocaine HCl	+	local anesthesia
epinephrine HCl	+	vasoconstriction (for local anesthesia)

new technique of fluoride iontophoresis that overcame any obstacles to its adoption.[24]

The drug of choice for aphthous ulcers or other nonspecific inflammatory conditions of oral mucosa is a steroid. This is indicated in Conn's Current Therapy (1975), which gives prominence to topical, or systemic steroid therapy. Yet dentists have not been satisfied with local therapy, and systemic steroids are fraught with dangers. The problem can be solved by applying the charged steroid, methyl prednisolone sodium succinate, by iontophoresis. This technique increases the penetration of the steroid locally, eliminating danger of side effects.

The drug of choice for herpes simplex virus (HSV) is idoxuridine (IDU). This drug has been used on humans for about 20 years, for HSV infections of the eye.[55] Although IDU does not possess any obvious site of charge, the author and his colleagues[19] showed that IDU penetration into skin could be greatly increased by either positive or negative iontophoresis.

The conditions to be treated must be near or at a body surface. Hypersensitive teeth, aphthous ulcers, herpes labialis, and mucosal pain can all be treated by iontophoresis because these conditions are localized at surfaces of the body.

Characteristics of the Active Electrode
(treatment electrode)

The charge of the drug determines the charge of the active electrode. The drug is propelled into the tissues by electronic repulsion. Therefore, negative ions are applied at the negative electrode (cathode), and positive ions at the positive electrode (anode). The outline above contains the important dental drugs, their polarity and the conditions for which they are used (see Table 8).

The active electrode must conform closely in size and shape to the tissue under treatment. Close adaptation of electrode to tissue is obtained by placing a cotton, paper or foam support containing the drug over the entire lesion. Since adaptation of electrodes to tissue is a formidable problem in the oral cavity, the author had to devise various novel means of electrode adaptation (see Chapter 11).

Characteristics of the Indifferent Electrode (return or dispersive)

An indifferent electrode is placed at any other site of the body. This electrode is opposite in charge to the active one, and contains any indifferent electrolyte. The volar surface of the forearm is a convenient site for the indifferent electrode and either sodium nitrate or sodium chloride is acceptable as an indifferent electrolyte. For patient comfort, the indifferent electrode should be at least as large in area as the active electrode.

Characteristics of the Power Source

It has been found that a DC power source delivering up to 27 volts is adequate for all uses in dentistry. Power sources delivering only 6 to 9 volts are underpowered and therefore inadequate. The power source may be 1) a safe, DC rectifier, 2) a rechargeable 9V battery with a step-up DC transformer, or 3) a conveniently replaceable 9V battery with a step-up DC transformer.

It is the author's experience that many dentists become discouraged with battery-operated iontophoresors because of inadequate power (lack of a step-up transformer) or decomposition of the battery (resulting in total loss of power when needed). The solution to the problem of battery decomposition is to use either a rechargeable (Nicad) battery or a unit which rejects when the battery is low. In any event, an adequate power source is the basis of the author's new technique for iontophoresis. Power supplies available for dental iontophoresis will be discussed in great detail in Chapter 10.

Characteristics of Current Flow

The current is allowed to flow between the electrodes, at or below the patient's sensory threshold. Discomfort is avoided by slowly increasing the rheostat on the power source and by never exceeding the patient's sensory threshold.

Current flow rate is measured in milliamperes (mA). The mA required for the dental procedures is described in Section III (treatment protocols).

The duration of current flow is set by a timer and is determined by the condition under treatment (see specific treatment protocols in Section III.

Current dosage is measured in mA times minutes (mA-min). The proper current dosage is obtained by first setting the mA and then setting duration to give the appropriate mA-min called for in the protocol for each procedure (see specific protocols in Section III).

Electrical Laws

There are only a few physical laws that are important in dental iontophoresis. Ohm's Law states that:

$$V = IR;$$

that is, electromotive force, V (in volts) equals current, I (in amps) times resistance, R (in ohms). The importance of Ohm's Law is that, at constant voltage (rheostat setting), any change in resistance results in a change in current level. Very often, the resistance decreases during a procedure; as a result, the mA will increase. This requires adjustment of the rheostat which is an annoyance and an interference with accurate dosing. Further, if the electrical dosage increases, there may be a danger to the tooth, or discomfort to the patient may result. Therefore, constant current during the procedures is a desirable attribute. A constant current compensator can be built into the power supply so that adjustments in rheostat setting are not required during the procedure.

Ohm's law is also useful in predicting that, in parallel circuits, more current will be carried by the pathway with less resistance. Thus, there is a need to insulate low resistance pathways to direct current flow into the desired tissue (see below: Insulation).

Coulomb's Law, a second law which has usefulness for dental iontophoresis, states that:

$$Q = IT;$$

that is, the quantity of electricity (Q) delivered is obtained by multiplying amperage (milliamps) times time, T (min). Thus, we state "mA-min" as the "current dosage," and each protocol states a recommended mA-min dosage and/or maximum. When stated as a maximum, mA-min (or maximum mA) must be observed to prevent damage to the tooth or other tissues.

A third electrical law of importance in dental iontophoresis is Faraday's Law, which states:

$$D = \frac{IT}{1Z1F}$$

or the amount of drug delivered, D (in gm-equivalents) equals current (I) times time (T), divided by valence (1Z1) times Faraday's Constant (F). The dentist is not required to manipulate this formula, but only to understand its significance: the more electricity delivered, the more drug delivered. Thus, we speak of electrical dosage and drug dosage in terms of mA-min.

Insulation and Shunting of Current

Up to the time of the author's work, insulation in dental iontophoresis was never considered. It is no wonder that many dentists gave up on iontophoresis! If one wishes to cause current entry into teeth, the soft tissues must be insulated. Also, if a dentin lesion is near a metal restoration, the metal must be insulated. Soft tissues, salivary films, and metal restorations all act as low resistance current sinks. Since the dentin is relatively high in resistance, parallel pathways of current flow are formed

and the most current will go through the low resistance pathway. The current carries the drug into the tissues, so that any short circuiting through low resistance pathways will detract greatly from the desired therapeutic effect. It has been found that masking tape, soft wax or Copalite[R] will adequately insulate metal restorations. Also a rubber dam or proper placement of the plastic electrode tips (so as to seal the gingiva) will insulate the soft tissue. Cotton rolls and vacuum are important for keeping the field dry and preventing saliva contamination of the electrode tip as well as build up of salivary films which may shunt the current.

Table 5 shows some resistances measured in dental tissues and materials. The significance of these measurements is related to the shape of the oral electrode and insulation as described in the following items.

1. It will be difficult to treat enamel because of shunting of current into dentin, even if the gingiva is isolated by a rubber dam. Therefore, treatment of enamel will require insulation from all other tissues, including dentin. The treatment of enamel is still in the experimental stages.

2. It is fairly easy to treat dentin lesions, provided the gingiva is isolated. Contact of electrode to enamel and dentin is satisfactory because most of the current goes into dentin.

3. The electrode tip must never contact dentin and metal because the metal will shunt almost all of the current. It follows that any sensitive dentin under a restoration or crown can only be treated before placing the restoration, or after removal of the restoration.

4. Sometimes, a compromise must be made when the electrode tip will touch dentin and soft tissue (as when the

brush technique is used). In such a case, we may increase the current dosage in proportion to the amount of shunting (for example, if the electrode is 50% on dentin and 50% on soft tissue, the mA-min can be at least doubled).

5. Masking tape, or soft wax, is used to insulate metal restorations. A rubber dam or the tygon tubing edge is used to insulate gingiva.

6. In tray techniques, the main insulation is obtained by contacting an insulator to the gingiva. When treating multiple hypersensitivities of uncut teeth, an alginate impression is made. The alginate serves as a good conductor but the gingiva must be insulated by placement of a rubber dam. If a rubber or silicone impression of cut preparations is available, it can be used to form the tray electrode because the gingiva can be adequately insulated by contact with nonconductive material. (Tray techniques will be covered in detail in Chapter 13.)

Table 5 Resistances of Dental Tissues and Materials*

Tissue or material	Resistance (K ohms)
Sound enamel	200-800
Defective enamel	less than 50
Dentin	less than 30
Cut dentin (oozing fluid)	2-3
Electrolyte (saliva)	2-3
Skin	6-9
Oral Mucosa	3-6
Metal restoration	0.1
Alginate	2
Silicone or rubber	∞
Acrylic	∞
Wax (nonconductive)	∞
Rubber dam	∞
Tygon tubing (electrode tip)	∞

*Unreported measurements made in Dr. Gangarosa's laboratory.
∞-infinity.

Electrical Safety

Iontophoresis is exceptionally safe when a modern system such as the Electro-Applicator System ™ is used. There is no electrical hazard to the patient, because of battery operation. In the author's opinion, there is no reason to use line-operated iontophoresors, even though they can be built with adequate safety features.

One should *certainly* throw away all line-operated units that are improperly grounded (having two-pronged plugs), or having a metal chassis! Connecting a patient to this type of unit is courting disaster. We should all be aware that electrical equipment does not mix with water. This is especially true of line-operated units. Do not use them near water! Better yet, don't use them at all!

Direct current can be damaging to tissues and therefore can cause burns. In over 500 tests of iontophoresis on skin of human volunteers, the author has had only 5 minor burns all of which were due to some fault in the operation. Burns are avoided as follows:

1. Respect the patient's threshold; if the patient feels discomfort, disconnect and check all systems before reconnecting;
2. Do not exceed the current levels described in the protocols;

3. Never let metal contact tissue; the tissues are always connected by a support of moistened paper, cotton or micropore foam;
4. Keep electrodes moist during procedures; and
5. Do not apply return electrode to an open wound or damaged tissue.

The author believes that many physicians became discouraged with iontophoresis because of poor technology, with the possibility of burns or other safety hazards. Those who espouse iontophoresis in medicine sometimes attempt to push the technique beyond its safety limits by recommending current levels exceeding one mA per square cm. This is a safe level of current in most tissues but may be dangerous to a fragile tissue, such as the cornea. Iontophoresis in ophthalmology was recommended at a level of 2 mA per eye,[94] and for dermatological use at 20-40 mA.[2] These levels would surely cause burns and discomfort, and result in condemnation of the method by physicians, dentists and patients.

Because pulpal safety is so important for dental practice, it will be considered in detail in Chapter 9.

Shocks

Shocks are avoided by connecting the patient with the rheostat setting at zero. If one connects the patient with the rheostat in the advanced position, the patient may be shocked. Thus, if you wish to temporarily stop the procedure and then reconnect, you must turn the rheostat back to zero. Also, the unit must be returned to the *off* position after each use in order to avoid connecting the next patient in the advanced rheostat position.

The modern ElectroApplicator™ system eliminates this shock problem, by means of a reject circuit. The unit will reject any attempt to connect the patient with the rheostat in the advanced position.

Shocks caused by dental iontophoresors are not a very great problem since they are usually slight to mild in terms of discomfort, but it is best to avoid them or the patient may become apprehensive.

Other Factors Which May Detract from Iontophoresis

1. Competing ions
Electrical current is carried by positive and negative ions in solution. There is no major distinction between ions of the same charge even though they are composed of different chemical elements. For example, positive current is carried by either sodium ions or lidocaine-hydrogen ions. However, since the mobility of sodium is greater than lidocaine, there is a greater preference for sodium to carry current. Therefore, solutions for iontophoresis should be as pure as possible and generally contain as few extraneous substances as possible. The author has recommended drug solutions prepared with ultrapure (distilled or de-ionized) water for maximum effectiveness of iontophoresis. Usually a suitable medication can be found to accommodate the maintenance of satisfactory solution purity. The dentist should closely follow the treatment protocols (Section III) in order to avoid drug solutions which contain competing ions.

2. Inactivation of drugs by tissues
If a drug reacts with protein causing subsequent inactivation, it will be difficult to use this drug by iontophoresis. For example, it is well known that copper ion inactivates molds and fungi in pure culture,[32] but is ineffective in the presence of con-

taminating protein. Therefore, iontophoresis of copper ion for fungal infections of the skin is doomed to failure because as the copper enters the tissues it is inactivated by host protein. Many physicians become discouraged with iontophoresis because of the ineffectiveness of copper in fungal disease (personal observation). We could predict similar failure of quaternary ammonium ions (for antibacterial effect) which also react with tissue proteins and become inactivated.

3. *Preservatives and other adjuvants*

Many solutions for parenteral use contain preservatives and other substances. We reported that preservatives will reduce the conductivity of solutions;[27] however, the effect of the preservatives in low concentrations is not great enough to detract from iontophoresis since only a 5-10% reduction of conductivity was noted. There usually remains enough conductivity of the drug so that current will be conducted by drug ions.

Summary

When iontophoresis is based upon sound scientific principle and logic, it will be successful. The new technology developed by the author eliminates possible pitfalls in dental iontophoresis, making it a safe and effective therapeutic tool to help the dentist treat patients who are in discomfort and who were previously neglected because no treatment was available.

Chapter 8

Diagnostic Aspects of Dentin Hypersensitivity

Our eyes are often blinded to observation of diseases for which we have no treatment! Dentists are taught to carefully diagnose dental caries for which adequate restorative treatments have been developed. Dentists are taught to be aware of periodontal disease and use their skills in corrective surgery. Dentists are taught to carefully consider the diagnosis of pulpitis because endodontic therapy depends upon proper diagnosis.

Dentin exposure which is not treatable by standard restorative procedures receives little attention. Patients suffer due to cervical dentin exposure, exposed root surfaces, occlusal wear and other causes. Patients afflicted with these problems are often not able to tolerate any change of temperature in their mouths and are victims of severe discomfort.

When a case of dentin hypersensitivity (which is not treatable by the usual corrective therapy) is noted, the dentist will probably either recommend a desensitizing toothpaste or attempt often tried, but usually ineffective, in-office treatments. Although none of these methods are consistently effective, the dentist is often pacified, in that he has performed the "accepted therapy," while the patient resigns himself to a life of discomfort. A further outcome of the encounter is that the victim will probably become a poor dental patient.

Fluoride iontophoresis, by the new technology described in this monograph, gives the dental profession an effective treatment for dentin hypersensitivity. In order to take maximum advantage of iontophoretic therapy, we need to consider the diagnostic aspects of dentin hypersensitivity. With better diagnosis and effective therapy, the patient will be better served and the dentist's armamentarium will be adequate to provide this additional therapy. If the dentist accepts fluoride iontophoresis for dentin hypersensitivity, his eyes will be opened to the many possibilities for usefulness. The dentist who adopts fluoride iontophoresis will be adequately rewarded both monetarily and in the quality of his practice. Accurate diagnosis will open the door to proper therapy by iontophoresis.

The diagnostic aspects of dentin hypersensitivity will be considered under the headings outlined in the following list.

1. Sensory Mechanism in Teeth
2. Oral Stimuli Causing Dentinal Sensation
3. Causes of Dental Pain
4. Differential Diagnosis of Dentin Hypersensitivity and its Therapeutic Prognosis
5. Diagnostic Procedures for Dentin Hypersensitivity

Sensory Mechanism in Teeth

All dentists and most dental patients can attest to an active sensory mechanism in teeth. The enamel and healthy periodontium, acting as insulators, protect the teeth from noxious stimuli. Under these conditions, the patient may be aware of hot and cold in his mouth, but there is no discomfort or pain. If the enamel protection is lost or if periodontal recession occurs, dentin may be exposed. Now the oral environment is directly in contact with the sensitive tissues. Now the patient may experience unusual discomfort due to changes in the oral environment. The patient has a problem which, if left unattended, can only deteriorate. Thus, it is the dentist's responsibility to give careful consideration to diagnosis and effective therapy.

Since dentin exposure leads to dentinal pain, the mechanism of transfer of pain from dentin to nerve is of interest. A recent monograph,[9] gathered a group of dental scientists together to discuss the subject. A full discussion is beyond the scope of this chapter, but a brief summary follows: 1) changes in the oral environment are detected by odontoblastic processes or within their tubules; 2) there is a transfer of information between odontoblastic process and nerve, probably near the odontoblastic cell (in the predentin); and 3) the pulpal nerves are activated to transmit the sensation of pain to the brain. Brännström and Aström[8] believe that the stimulus is transferred to the nerve by osmotic changes within the dentinal tubules, the so-called "Hydrodynamic Effect." If this be accepted, then any therapy which will block the dentinal tubules will have an effect to reduce dentinal pain and the duration of effect will be dependent upon the permanence of the block.

There is recent evidence that fluoride ion may block the dentinal tubules by precipitation of calcium fluoride from intratubular fluid which is supersaturated with respect to calcium and fluoride ions.[13,91] Since iontophoresis results in penetration deeply into the tubules,[59] one would expect that precipitation in the tubules would be enhanced when fluoride iontophoresis is performed.

Although Lefkowitz[59,60] claimed that the mechanism of iontophoresis involves formation of massive amounts of reparative dentin within the pulp canal, the author believes that fluoride iontophoresis acts too rapidly for the reparative dentin mechanism to be plausible as an explanation. Furthermore, Walton et al.[17] reported that 1mA-min or 5 mA-min of current applied by fluoride iontophoresis to exposed root dentin of dog caused no changes in odontoblasts, pulp or dentin after 7 days or 80 days (see Chapter 9). Thus, the mechanism of fluoride iontophoresis which causes dentin desensitization is not established and is open for study.

Oral Stimuli Causing Dentinal Pain

After the dentin is exposed, it may repair itself by calcification,[42] the tubular spaces may be blocked by being clogged with debris[74] or the tubules may remain wide open.[74] It is probably the latter situation which results in dentin hypersensitivity, since wide open tubular spaces would be conducive to passage of stimuli.[50] Such a state may favor dentin conduction of stimuli due to temperature changes (cold and hot), chemical changes (sugar, osmotic effects, acrid chemical) or touch.

Causes of Dentinal Pain

As discussed above, dentinal pain results from direct contact of exposed dentin with the oral environment. Pain may be due to the following sensory stimuli:

temperature changes
  cold
  heat
chemical changes
  sugar
  osmotic changes
  acrid chemicals (acids, etc.)
touch

Plaque may contribute to the problem because of acid decalification caused by bacterial acid production and the formation of toxic products which may diffuse through the tubules and cause pulpal irritation.

Pulpal irritation may also result from constant bombardment of stimuli from the hypersensitive dentin; if no treatment is instituted the pulp may become inflamed which results in further hyperemia leading to pulpal changes which, in turn can result in a longer lasting pain with a tendency toward irreversible pulpitis. Following chronic inflammation, the pulp becomes irreversibly altered requiring root canal therapy.

Our efforts should be to treat dentin hypersensitivity in the stage before inflammation of the pulp becomes irreversible. The pulp can endure many insults, but as long as the pain is transient, the prognosis for iontophoretic fluoride therapy is favorable. When the pain begins to endure beyond the application of the stimulus, the prognosis becomes less favorable. Needless to say, when the stage of chronic inflammation and hyperemia results in pulpal pressure and necrotic changes, the prognosis for iontophoretic therapy becomes extremely unfavorable.

If there is any question about the prognosis, it would be worthwhile to try iontophoretic fluoride therapy; if this fails root canal therapy can then be performed. As a matter of fact, the author, in collaboration with endodontists, has found fluoride iontophoresis to be a useful diagnostic tool in

endodontics; i.e., any tooth which does not respond favorably to fluoride iontophoresis may be best treated by root canal therapy. Since many dentists have a problem deciding when to do a root canal, this diagnostic tool would be a helpful aid to dental practice.

Differential Diagnosis of Dentin Hypersensitivity and Its Therapeutic Prognosis

The following list of causes of dental pain should be considered in the differential diagnosis.

1. Dental caries
2. Exposed root surface (recession or iatrogenic)
3. Cervical erosion
4. Abrasion or wear (natural or iatrogenic)
5. Enamel hypoplasia
6. Malformation at cementoenamel junction (CEJ)
7. Occlusal traumatism
8. Pulpitis
9. Pulpal abscess
10. Cracked tooth
11. Improperly insulated restoration

Each item in the above list will be reviewed in terms of iontophoretic therapy.

1. Dental caries

Once the enamel protection is lost due to decalcification, the dentin becomes exposed. Many patients become extremely sensitive to temperature or chemical changes at the time when dentin is first exposed. Complaints of sensitivity in a tooth or quadrant should be carefully studied by examination with X-ray, explorer and other diagnostic tools. All carious teeth should be restored, with adequate insulation, in order to eliminate dental caries from the differential diagnosis and relieve sensitivity due to this cause.

2. Exposed root surface

During aging, the periodontal tissues gradually recede exposing the root surfaces to the oral environment. Root surfaces may also be exposed during corrective surgery for periodontal disease. The cementum layer is easily lost due to abrasion by toothbrushing or during root planing. Thus, root exposure inevitably exposes root dentin.

Dentin hypersensitivity following root exposure is readily treated by iontophoresis of fluoride ion. For massive exposure, following corrective periodontal therapy, the author has developed the tray technique for treating multiple hypersensitivities (see Chapter 13).

3. Cervical erosion

Cervical erosion is a common finding; many patients have eroded areas in the buccal, gingival areas. Such erosions are probably related to acid attack either from plaque or due to acid foods. Very often abrasion from toothbrushing or from lip pressure contributes to the problem. In fact, some authors attribute cervical exposure of dentin to a combination of acid attack and abrasive forces.

The prognosis for treating cervical dentin exposure by fluoride iontophoresis is extremely favorable and the author has experienced a success rate of over 95% of cases treated.

4. Abrasion or wear

Abrasion is noted on the buccal surfaces of teeth especially in association with toothbrushing. If the patient has an anterior to posterior scrubbing habit, the grooves created may be several millimeters deep. Abrasive substances in the diet or in chewing materials (tobacco, snuff, etc.) may result in occlusal wear. Also, night grinding or clenching of the teeth may cause wearing of the enamel. Sometimes enamel wear may be so severe that the subject's teeth are worn to the gingival margin (Fig. 16). The dentist may also expose dentin in occlusal equilibration or in rest preparation for removable prosthesis. The prognosis for fluoride iontophoresis treatment of occlusal wear or abraded areas is very favorable (over 95% success).

5. Enamel hypoplasia

Enamel hypoplasia may result in frank exposure of dentin or in reduced enamel unable to perform its insulating function. In either case, the teeth may be highly sensitive to temperature changes. The author has treated two bicuspids in one child, who was referred by the Chairman of Pedodontics at the Medical College of Georgia. This 12-year-old boy had been unable to eat ice cream, hot soup or place anything in the mouth which caused a temperature change. He was also an uncooperative patient because the vacuum or water spray caused extreme discomfort. Fluoride iontophoresis was performed, with immediate relief. The child then became a cooperative dental patient and experienced the joy of ice cream and just plain cold water for the first time in his life.

The prognosis for treating enamel hypoplasia is extremely promising but further study is required to evaluate the degree of success, since only one case (involving two teeth) has been treated. Furthermore, if the dentin is not exposed, fluoride iontophoresis may not be useful unless the enamel is extremely thin.

Further study of the value of fluoride iontophoresis in enamel hypoplasia is indicated.

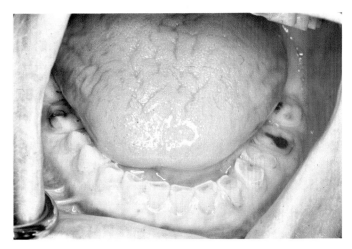

Fig. 16 Massive abrasion of the teeth. The patient was a tobacco chewer and had worn many lower teeth almost to the gingiva. There were no pulp exposures, but the dentin was extremely sensitive. One fluoride iontophoresis treatment with the tray technique (see Chapter 13) restored normal sensitivity.

6. *Malformation at the cemento-enamel junction (CEJ)*

Malformation of the CEJ exposes dentin in the gingival area. It is rather rare and occurs usually in the bicuspid-cuspid area. When the subject has CEJ malformation, the dentin can be excruciatingly sensitive to heat, cold and explorer touch.

The author has had extremely good success in treating the CEJ malformation by fluoride iontophoresis.

7. *Occlusal traumatism*

The tooth can become extremely sensitive due to traumatic effects of a high spot. This condition usually affects the periodontal membrane but sometimes the pulp is involved. Occlusal traumatism is best treated by occlusal equilibration and the fluoride iontophoresis should not be used unless dentin is exposed. If the tooth is sensitive to percussion, the high spot must be eliminated in preference to any other treatment.

8. *Pulpitis*

If the tooth has pulpitis with dentin exposure, the fluoride iontophoresis of a dentin lesion may be helpful. If no dentin exposure is noted, there is no indication for fluoride iontophoresis.

The author has had several cases of extreme pain while drilling to perform a pulpectomy, which were facilitated by iontophoresis of fluoride into the dentinal covering over the pulp. These patients could not tolerate drilling on the dentin even under local anesthesia. Following fluoride iontophoresis (one mA for 15 min.), comfortable extirpation of the pulp was possible.

9. *Pulpal abscess*

Any pain due to pulpal abscess must be treated by standard root canal therapy. Fluoride iontophoresis is not rationale for abscessed teeth. Drainage is the treatment of choice.

10. *Cracked tooth*

A cracked tooth causing dental pain must be treated by standard therapy including endodontic, periodontic and restorative measures. Iontophoresis of fluoride does not appear to be permanently helpful for a cracked tooth since the pain arises from the pulp and not from exposed dentin. Relief of pain caused by fluoride iontophoresis in a cracked tooth is only temporary.

11. Improperly insulated restoration

This is one of the major problems of restorative dentistry. A filled, or crowned tooth in which a temperature change occurs in the mouth, results in an irritating situation for both patient and dentist. Usually the patient suffers with this problem for many years because the dentist insists that the discomfort will "go away" with time. And "go away" it will! Either nature will cause reparative dentin formation to heal the insult or the pulp will "give-up" requiring endodontic therapy.

The author has had a great amount of success eliminating sensitivity of crown and bridge preparations, deep cavities, or thermally uncomfortable restorations by using fluoride iontophoresis on the exposed dentin before restoration was attempted or after removal of the restoration. If the tooth is restored, the restoration must be removed in order to re-expose the dentin before performing the fluoride iontophoresis. By anticipating this problem, the dentist can use fluoride iontophoresis to prevent development of thermal discomfort, saving himself and the patient a great deal of trouble. The author uses fluoride iontophoresis on any preparation that is excessively sensitive to a cold air blast (rating of 3 or 4 on the discomfort scale). Also, the author believes that all crowns and bridges should be cemented without anesthesia; fluoride iontophoresis of the exposed dentin makes this possible.

In the case of permanently cemented crowns or bridges, the author has had good results using a brush technique (see Chapter 13) around the margins, providing there is dentin exposure at the margins, as indicated by the air-blast test.

Diagnostic Procedures for Dentin Hypersensitivity

Diagnosis is always fundamental in arriving at the proper and indicated therapy; a well conceived treatment plan which is well understood by both patient and dentist is a necessity. During all entry examinations for new patients and on recall, the patient should be questioned concerning tooth hypersensitivity. The examination should include not only a questionnaire, but also the air-blast test on several teeth to determine the presence of sensitivity. When tooth hypersensitivity is apparent, the problem must be further explored to determine its cause and the location of the dentinal lesions. The dentist may find teeth that are non-carious but still hypersensitive to oral stimuli. Any hypersensitive teeth can be rated by procedures described below and the therapy required can be added to the treatment plan. Fluoride iontophoresis can now be instituted for hypersensitive teeth, resulting in improved dental therapy which relieves discomfort and prevents the onset of further problems during other forms of therapy. Further, the development of an adequate treatment plan allows the dentist to provide fluoride iontophoresis on a fee-for-service basis. The author believes that many problems of dentin hypersensitivity following restorations or periodontal surgery can be avoided by instituting these diagnostic procedures. No case should be started until all hypersensitivity is under control. By anticipating this problem, the dentist saves himself and his patients much discomfort and anxiety.

The diagnostic procedures for detecting dentin hypersensitivity will now be described.

1. Air blast

The tooth to be tested is isolated from the

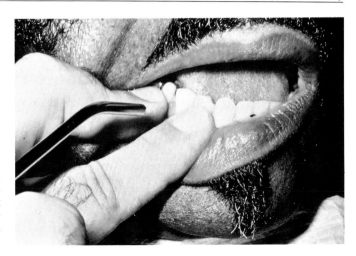

Fig. 17 Diagnosis of thermal hypersensitivity. A one second air blast is directed at the suspected surface, while adjacent teeth are covered with the fingers. For further details, see text.

other teeth by appropriately placing cotton rolls, or the examiner's fingers (Fig. 17). The air syringe is then placed close to the suspected area and the button depressed while the operator counts "1-1000." The patient is asked to rate the discomfort on the following discomfort scale:

0—no discomfort
1—mild discomfort
2—moderate discomfort
3—severe discomfort (transient)
4—intolerable discomfort
   (lasting after the stimulus)

This scale is not considered quantitative but rather is a guide to the patients' subjective and relative perception of discomfort. However, the author has found that the patient can reproduce these ratings quite well.

The author treats all teeth rated 2 or higher, starting with the highest rated teeth at the first appointment. The ratings are recorded both before and after treatment on an appropriate form (see Fig. 18). The author's group has found that about 85-90% of teeth, rated 3 or 4 before treatment, are rated 0 or 1 immediately after treatment and on successive appointments for up to

10 years (the longest period of follow-up for this method). Treated teeth remain healthy and have vital electric pulp tests as long as they have been followed.

About 10-15% of teeth require a second treatment, in the author's experience. Teeth which are still hypersensitive after the first treatment (rated 2 or higher) are retreated one week later (see Chapter 9, Pulpal Safety), at which time a comfortable rating (0 or 1) almost invariably results. Rarely, a third treatment is needed. There are only a few cases, less than 5%, that are resistant to this treatment, but the percentage of successes make fluoride iontophoresis a valuable in-office therapy for hypersensitive dentin.

2. Cold water

Some patients are hypersensitive but the air blast does not give a high discomfort rating. A more rigorous test is to squirt 0.2 ml of ice water directly on the suspected area. This test is also excellent for detecting sensitivity under a metal restoration and is therefore, useful in distinguishing between the latter and exposed dentin lesion. (For treating sensitive dentin under a restoration, the dentin must be re-ex-

Diagnostic Form For Dentin Hypersensitivity

Name _____ Date _____

Rating

Tooth #	Status (DMF)	1st Treatment before	1st Treatment after	2nd Treatment before	2nd Treatment after	Tooth #	Status (DMF)	1st Treatment before	1st Treatment after	2nd Treatment before	2nd Treatment after
1						17					
2						18					
3						19					
4						20					
5						21					
6						22					
7						23					
8						24					
9						25					
10						26					
11						27					
12						28					
13						29					
14						30					
15						31					
16						32					

DMF: D = decayed; M = missing; F = filled.
Test used: air blast (1 second; count 1-1,000)
cold water (0.2 ml ice water, rapidly on each area)
explorer touch
rinse: cold water or grapefruit juice
Ratings: 0 = normal sensation; 1 = mild discomfort; 2 = moderate;
3 = severe, transient; 4 = severe, intolerable.

Figure 18

posed). The same discomfort rating scale (0-4) is used in the cold water test as in the air-blast test. Results of treatment by iontophoresis have been similar, irrespective of the stimulus used for testing.

3. Grapefruit juice

If the patient responds more to acrid chemicals that to thermal changes, then grapefruit juice (from a can) may be substituted for the cold water. Discomfort ratings are similar to those described for cold-air blast, and results of fluoride iontophoresis are also similar when judged by this test.

4. Tolerance

One ounce of either cold tap water, ice water, or grapefruit juice is held in the mouth as long as possible before and after fluoride iontophoresis. (The selection of stimulus type is dependent upon patient sensitivity type and tolerance.) Many patients, who could not perform this test (zero tolerance), were able to hold the fluid in the mouth for 15 seconds or longer after the fluoride iontophoresis.

5. Intolerance to testing

If the patient is unable to tolerate the one-second air blast, giving several ratings "beyond 4," the test is discontinued, and testing is performed only after completion of fluoride iontophoresis.

6. Explorer touch

The explorer is firmly pressed across suspected sensitive areas. Again, discomfort ratings are from 0-4. Many patients who are not hypersensitive to cold are extremely sensitive to explorer touch. Sometimes this condition makes operative procedures difficult and some of these patients cannot tolerate scaling unless a local anesthetic is administered. Fluoride iontophoresis can aid patient cooperation and make dental practice more pleasant by relieving the touch sensitivity.

Chapter 9

Pulpal Safety of Fluoride Iontophoresis

This is an extremely important consideration for dentists. The dental pulp is one of the most sensitive organs, responding unfavorably to caustics and inflammatory agents with possible irreversible damages ending in pulpal necrosis. We would like our desensitization procedures to be non-irritating, and any resultant changes to be reversible. To this end, we recommend that no caustic chemicals nor physically damaging agents (for example, electrosurgical current) be applied to the dentin (see Chapter 8).

The safety of applying controlled amounts of direct current to the dentin was documented by Scott.[83] He recommended on the basis of his histological study, 1 mA-min of direct current as safe, causing no permanent injury. Scott believed that desensitization occurred without lowering pulp vitality. Lefkowitz[59] and Lefkowitz et al.[60] concluded that iontophoresis causes no irreversible injury to pulpal tissues.

Our study on pulpal safety in dogs[30] will now be considered in great detail because pulpal safety must be considered the single most important subject in any dental therapy.

Seventy-eight developing permanent teeth of two young adult, mongrel dogs were studied. Seven days after surgery to expose the roots, the periodontal pack was removed and the cementum was planed with periodontal curettes to expose cervical root dentin. Iontophoresis of sodium fluoride was applied to the exposed roots by a procedure similar to that used with humans.

Procedures were repeated to give observation periods of 7 and 80 days in each dog. Teeth were divided at random into experimental and control groups.

1. Experimental
   (a) Fluoride ion at therapeutic dosage (0.5 mA. for 2 minutes).
   (b) Fluoride ion at high current dosage (1.0 mA. for 5 minutes).
2. Negative controls
   (a) Unexposed, untreated teeth.
   (b) Root exposure alone.
   (c) Fluoride ion, topical application.
   (d) Current dosage alone.
3. Positive controls
   Exposed root surfaces were ground with a diamond fissure bur in an air-turbine handpiece without water coolant. This procedure was designed to cause an inflammatory response in the underlying pulp, providing a comparison with the experimental teeth.

The mineralizing front of dentin was marked at intervals by tetracycline injection at the time of the original surgical procedure and at the time of the experimental procedure, (7 days later). Another bone marker (Procion brilliant red) was injected

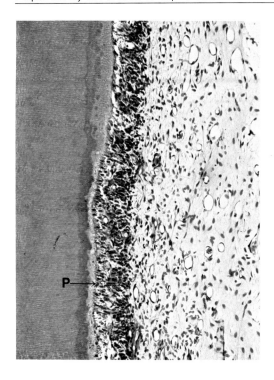

Fig. 19 Photomicrograph of Dog's Tooth after Grinding Without Coolant (Positive Control after 7 days). Pulp-dentin region underlying tubules extending from a ground region. In response to the grinding, the odontoblast layer has been disrupted. Inflammatory cells have infiltrated the subodontoblast and odontoblast zones. In some regions, the predentin (P) is markedly narrowed. (Original magnification, x270.)

intraperitoneally, 14 days after the surgery. Therefore, relative amounts of dentin formed following the procedures could be determined by measuring and comparing the amount of dentin formed in experimental and control specimens.

Throughout the observation period, the teeth of both dogs were brushed three times weekly to minimize plaque accumulation. The dogs were sacrificed and portions of each tooth were obtained for histologic, electron microscopic and visual examination. Central pulp and subodontoblastic zones were examined histologically for inflammation, cell disruption, hemorrhage, or vasodilation. Odontoblastic layers were examined with light and electron microscopy for the presence of gross or fine structural aberration. Within the same tooth, areas of dentin beneath exposed and treated root surfaces were compared to areas of dentin beneath enamel for evidence of morphologic aberrations and alterations in the rate of formation.

Of all the groups, only the positive controls (treated by grinding without water coolant) of both 7- and 80-day specimens demonstrated histologic alterations of the pulp and dentin. After 7 days (Fig. 19), the odontoblast layer was disrupted, the predentin narrowed, and the subodontoblastic zone showed inflammatory cells. After 80 days (specimen not shown), there appeared to be complete recovery; there was an intact layer of odontoblasts.

There were no differences noted between negative controls (Fig. 20) and experimental specimens (Fig. 21) for either the 7- or 80-day observation period. The regions of pulp underlying root surfaces, which were denuded and then iontophoresed, were

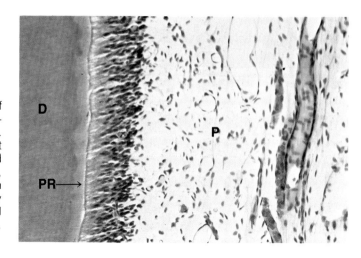

Fig. 20 Photomicrograph of untreated dog's tooth. (Negative Control after 7 or 8 days). Odontoblast layer and adjacent pulp (P) and predentin (PR) and dentin (D) from the unexposed, untreated control. This tooth has not been subjected to any experimental procedures, and the tissues appear normal. (Original magnification, x280.)

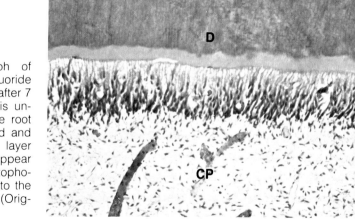

Fig. 21 Photomicrograph of dog's tooth treated by fluoride iontophoresis, 5 mA-min, after 7 days. This area of pulp is underlying the region of the root surface that was exposed and treated. The odontoblast layer and central pulp (CP) appear unaffected by fluoride iontophoresis and appear similar to the control pulp in Figure 20. (Original magnification x280.)

not altered. There were no differences between low (therapeutic) and high (five times therapeutic) current levels. Also, only the positive controls (ground teeth) showed accelerated dentin formation. By contrast, the negative controls and iontophoresed specimens had similar patterns of dentinogenesis.

Neither the current alone, nor in combination with sodium fluoride, appeared to alter the rate of dentin formation.

In summary, iontophoresis of sodium fluoride on surgically exposed and scaled root surfaces in dogs produced the following:

1. No demonstrable effect on odontoblasts at the histologic and ultrastructural level; this was true for both low and high current dosage levels for both 7- and 80-day observation periods.

2. No demonstrable effect of the electric current on the central pulp or subodontoblastic zone.

3. No apparent stimulation by iontophoresis of either primary or irritation dentin formation.

We concluded that either 1-mA-min or 5

mA-min of direct current electricity with 2% NaF is safe for pulpal tissue. Although the higher amount appears safe, we do not recommend exceeding 1 mA-min (on insulated teeth) so that the highest possible margin of safety is maintained.

In the author's clinical experience, there is no reason to lengthen the treatment time because the recommended 1 mA-min has been extremely effective. Further, it is difficult to raise the current level because the pain threshold is exceeded at about 0.5 mA. The author believes that pain during the procedure indicates tissue damage occurring. Therefore, he recommends that the sensory threshold not be exceeded. The maximum mA levels recommended in the protocols are controlled by our findings on sensory threshold.

As an added precaution, our dental practice, treatment protocols, recommend that repeat treatments be performed at 1 week intervals. This is to assure that any possible changes induced by the current are reversed before a second treatment is started.

Over a period of 10 years, the author has treated more than 1,000 teeth by fluoride iontophoresis; to his knowledge, none of the teeth treated has subsequently required a root canal. Many of the cases have been followed regularly by recall, and the treated teeth continue to remain vital, by electric pulp test.

This evidence indicates that fluoride iontophoresis is an exceptionally safe and biologically acceptable method of dentin desensitization.

Section III

Operating Instructions for Dental Iontophoresis

Chapter 10

Power Supplies Available

Line-operated Units

There are some iontophoresors being used which are operated through the 120 V AC wall outlet. The AC output is converted to DC by means of a rectifier. The author feels that line-operated units should not be used in dental practice because of safety considerations either real or imagined.

Any unit with a two-pronged plug should be discarded since this is a real safety hazard. The benefits of iontophoresis are not worth the risk of connecting an ungrounded patient to the AC line. Any attempts to use a makeshift ground should be discouraged.

There has been much experience with three-pronged plug-in units for pilocarpine iontophoresis in children. This diagnostic technique for cystic fibrosis is used daily on infants and children in almost every major medical center in the U.S.A. Many of the pilocarpine iontophoresors have safety-protected circuits with well-grounded, three pronged plugs. Some manufacturers are HTL, Inc., Lancer, Orion, etc. The author considers units with three-pronged plugs and safety-protected circuits as safe, since the chances of a hazard to the patient are extremely remote with proper grounding.

The author's first experience with iontophoresis in dental practice was with units adapted from the pilocarpine iontophoresis. During this research phase, the author realized that some of the earlier iontophoresors recommended for dentistry were underpowered. Therefore, he specified that his first dental iontophoresor would be a unit with a three-pronged plug and safety-protected circuit. The author coined the term "Electro-Medicator" to describe this system. He also specified a novel electrode system for oral application of drugs. Later, an additional margin of safety was added by specifying a rechargeable battery for the Electro-Medicator, Model C-1, power supply. The only advantage of battery operated units over the line-operated units is that an imagined risk may exist with the latter. For example, a patient with cardiac disease may think that there would be a hazard from being connected to the wall outlet, irrespective of the number of safety features incorporated into the unit. This source of annoyance is eliminated by using only battery-operated units in dentistry.

Simple Battery-operated Units (dry cell batteries)

Most dental iontophoresors used in the past (Chayes-Siemon) or currently available (Chayes-Siemon type or hand-held models) provide about 4-8 volts from a dry cell, battery source. This is considered inadequate since the dentin has a resistance up to 80,000 ohms; using Ohm's law, current (I) is equal to voltage (E) divided by resistance (R), the following can be derived:

E(volts)	R(ohms)	I(Amp)
8	80,000	0.0001
25	80,000	0.0003

I(mAmp)	Duration(min)	(mA-min)
0.1	10	1
0.3	3.3	1

The author's studies indicate that an electrical dose of one mA-min is safe for delivery to the tooth; since mA-min = current × duration, therefore, 0.3 mA must be applied for approximately 3.3 minutes to desensitize a tooth. Most teeth have dentin resistance less than 80,000 ohms so the 25 volt source is considered adequate for dental practice. The 4 to 8 volt source is inadequate because 10 min. or more of treatment time would be required.

Another problem with dry cell models is that the batteries decompose. The resultant loss of power may occur without any warning, resulting in frustration to the dentist when power is missing at a critical time. A warning light indicating the loss of power (as in Motion Control's Phoresor) resolves this problem, but this feature is not available in earlier models.

Rechargeable Power Source

The units originally recommended by the author for clinical dental practice contained rechargeable batteries. A 9 volt charger was used to keep a nickel-cadmium battery at full charge. A multiplier circuit increased the voltage to 25-27 volts. Ten hours of charging was required

to bring the battery up to full charge and the charge would hold for 5-7 days. The best policy was to keep the unit in a convenient place in the operatory with the charger plugged in during non-operation.

Figure 22 shows the face of a typical iontophoresis unit of this type. A is a milliammeter calibrated in 0.1 mA, with a maximum of 1 mA. B represents the output jacks labelled + and −, which are color-coded red and black, respectively. C is a power on-off switch, which serves as a rheostat, calibrated on a relative scale of 1-10. D is a pilot light which flashes when the power switch is on. E is the charging jack. When the charger is plugged in, the unit will not supply power. F is a timer and G is a timer switch. In the off-timer mode, the unit will supply power irrespective of the position of the timer. When the unit is operated in the on-timer mode, power will be cut off when the timer reaches zero. Because the timer on-off switch created some confusion in operation, it has been eliminated in the more advanced dental office power source.

An Advanced Power Supply for Dental Office Use

Figure 23 shows the Phoresor™ Model PM 600 by Motion Control, Inc. Salt Lake City. This power supply is the ultimate in a dental office iontophoresor. It is small and has an attractive chassis. Although the unit is powered by a 9 V replaceable battery, the circuitry converts the voltage through a step-up transformer to 45 volts DC. Also, a battery warning light is on the control panel, so that the dentist can replace the battery when indicated. Another convenient feature of the Phoresor is that an audible signal sounds when the battery is placed backwards into the battery receptacle.

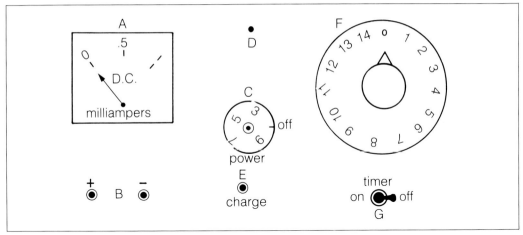

Fig. 22   Diagram of the author's first dental Iontophoresor (EA, C-1 or EM, A-1). (Actual unit shown in Fig. 5.): a) milliammeter, b) output jacks, c) power on-off switch, d) pilot light, e) charging jack, f) timer, g) timer switch.

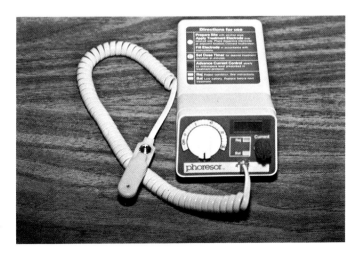

Fig. 23   The Phoresor™, model PM 600-2. A modern Iontophoresor for dental office use.

A most important innovation of the Phoresor is the constant-current supply. When the power supply has no constant-current feature, any resistance changes during the procedure require adjustment of the rheostat. Thus, when operating the older units (see below), someone had to constantly adjust the rheostat in order to be certain the correct mA and mA-min were attained. The Phoresor, by means of a constant-current control in the circuitry, automatically adjusts for any change in resistance in the external circuit during the procedure.

The digital readout of the Phoresor is another advantageous feature. This allows more accurate dosing, since one can only guess the exact mA reading on a needle-meter.

A further advantage of the Phoresor is the reject circuitry. A warning light is noted when the battery is low. Also, when the timer is in the *off* position, when the electrodes are improperly connected, and when the impedance of the outside circuit is either too low or too high, both a warning light and an audible signal can be noted. These warnings help the operator to deduce any problems with the set-up which would adversely affect the treatment.

The Phoresor will be discussed further in Chapter 12 (Operating Instructions for the ElectroApplicator System, Model C-2.)

Comparisons of Currently Available Power Supplies and Systems

Tables 6 and 7 indicate the characteristics of iontophoretic power sources and systems. In row 1, the characteristics of the Electro-Applicator System, Model C-2 (EAS,C-2) are listed. The EAS,C-2 is superior and the most dependable system compared to others currently available (rows 2, 3, 4). The Phoresor (EAS,C-2)

power unit has the highest power supply (45 V), a current limitor, a dependable source of energy (disposable batteries), constant-current feature, excellent provision for insulation, digital display, the most adaptable electrode system, fixed disposable return electrode, low potential for shocks and burns, and reject features (which indicate improper procedures to the operator). This system is readily available, highly reliable, and has good service and support. Because of its dependability, the cost of the EAS,C-2 can be easily recovered in services rendered to patients.

The ElectroMedicator A-1 (EM,A-1) and the ElectroApplicator C-1 (EA,C-1) are almost equivalent in performance. The EA,C-1 has been discontinued because of the introduction of the more advanced EAS,C-2. EM,A-1 has been rather difficult to obtain, in the author's experience. Also, EM,A-1, was designed in 1975 and has not been changed to meet the author's latest specifications. Additional problems with EM,A-1 include:1) rechargeable battery circuit caused some difficulties; 2) no constant-current circuit; 3) difficulty in reading the exact mA; 4) electrode system has not been changed for maximum adaptability; 5) return electrode has too many parts; 6) high chance for shocks; and 7) no reject features.

The Chayes-Siemon type-units were not well conceived on a physical, electrical basis. The power source is too weak and there is no indicator to warn of low charge. The current is voltage-limited (not enough EMF supplied), and there is no provision for a constant-current. The meter is not well calibrated. A brush electrode is supplied, as well as wires for a tray technique, but no provision for insulation is described. The return electrode is hand-held by the patient, which is not ideal. The patient can quite readily be shocked because of the lack of reject circuits. The au-

Table 6 Currently Available Dental Iontophoresis Systems

| | Battery | | Current | | Digital display? | Provision for insulation | Adapt-ability of electrodes |
	Rated EMF / Operating EMF	Type	Maximum	Constant?			
ElectroApplicator Model C-2 (EAS, C-2)	9V / up to 45V	disposable	2 mA (current limitor)	yes	yes	excellent	good
ElectroMedicator A-1, or Electro-Applicator C-1*	9V / up to 27V	rechargeable	2 mA (current limitor)	no	no	good	moderate
Chayes-Siemon Type	9V / 7-9V	disposable	voltage-limited	no	no	none	slight (brush & tray)
Hand-Held Models	4.5V / 3.5-4.5V	disposable	voltage-limited	no	no	none	none (brush only)

*EA, C-1, Discontinued

Table 7 (Continuation)

	Return electrode	Possibility of shocks	Reject feature?	Availability of service	Reliability	Cost	Overall rating
ElectroApplicator Model C-2	fixed, (disposable)	very low	yes	excellent	very high	reasonable ($600 +)	excellent
ElectroMedicator A-1, or ElectroApplicator C-1*	fixed, (assembly needed)	high	no	difficult*	high	reasonable ($400-500)	good
Chayes-Siemon Type	hand-held	high	no	difficult	low	medium ($160)	poor
Hand-Held Models	through dentist-patient contact	high	no	disposable(?)	very low	low ($40)	poor

*EA, C-1, Discontinued

thor found that these units were not readily available, and that battery replacement is not simple. Since the amount of power supplied by such units is low, the reliability is also low, accounting for the lack of general acceptance by dentists. Although the original cost is modest, the poor reliability makes this unit a poor investment.

The hand-held models, which are still being actively promoted, have very little merit. The cost is low, but the author considers these a waste of money and patients' and dentists' time. It is obvious, in Tables 6 and 7, that the hand-held models are poorly rated in each category.

Summary

The dentist should choose a power supply for iontophoresis which is safe and effective. Battery operated units are the safest. Effectiveness is obtained by using an adequately powered unit which supplies 25-45 V DC. The Dentelect ElectroApplicator Model C-1 is considered excellent. The Phoresor™ has been adopted by the author as the power supply for the Electro-Applicator System, Model C-2. The Phoresor™ by Motion Control, Inc. is considered the ultimate in a dental iontophoresor, incorporating many novel and helpful features. The Dentelect Electrode Set™ by LPG provides the electrode adaptability needed in a modern system.

Chapter 11

Accessories for Iontophoresors

The author's contributions, which made iontophoresis technically feasible in the dental office, are:

1. Specification of an adequate power supply;
2. Specification of a versatile system of electrode accessories to adapt to the oral cavity; and
3. Specification of use of insulation to prevent loss of current.

Dental iontophoresors which have not incorporated the modern accessories needed to adequately perform iontophoresis in dental practice include the 3M Ionator and Parkell's Desensitron.

The author's oral electrode accessories which can be obtained in a package, the Dentelect Electrode-Set™ by LPG are compared to other available accessories and are detailed in Chapter 12.

Return Electrode

The skin electrode for pilocarpine iontophoresis or any reasonable facsimile is satisfactory. The ElectroMedicator, Model A-1 (EM,A-1), used a black, plastic conductive disc manufactured to receive a banana-jack connector. The disc was covered by a thick piece of blotter paper which received the indifferent electrolyte; a celluloid cover surrounded the disc to insulate the skin. Recent models of EM,A-1 have been altered, using stainless steel for the conductive surface instead of conductive plastic. The use of stainless steel is to be discouraged because it deteriorates due to electrical current; also any metal ions generated would compete for the current and metal ions might deposit in the skin.

The return electrode which was part of the Dentelect ElectroApplicator, Model C-1 (Fig. 6b), was machined from non-conductive nylon or teflon and contained a wire screen within the plastic housing. Instead of a paper support, urethane foam pads were used as inserts in the plastic housing to hold the indifferent electrolyte. Depending upon the type of *return electrode* used, appropriate pads or paper covers and celluloid discs are needed. An electrode strap or band is needed to secure the *return electrode* in place on the forearm (Fig. 6a). Another more convenient form of the return electrode is a disposable band-aid configuration (Fig. 24). In the Electro-Applicator System, Model C-2 (EAS,C-2), the *return electrode* has a snap attachment which fits into the *output cable* of the Phoresor. Note the application and attachment of the *return electrode* to the Phoresor (Fig. 24). There are two types of return electrodes supplied in the EAS,C-2. When the drug to be applied at the *active elec-*

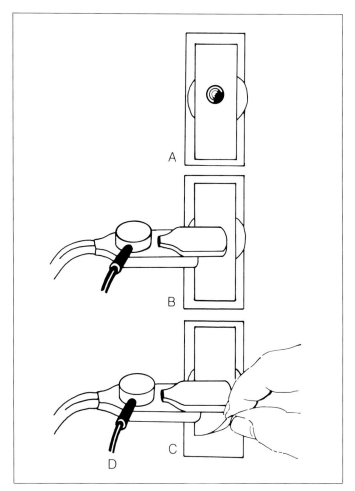

Fig. 24 Disposable return electrode: a) return electrode as supplied, b) return electrode attached to Phoresor terminal, c) removal of return electrode backing.

trode is negative (as for fluoride ion for the desensitization of hypersensitive teeth), the male snap (+) *return electrode* is attached to the *output cable*. If a positive drug is to be applied, a female snap (−) *return electrode* is selected. The *return electrode* is saturated with 1% sodium nitrate.

Two out-moded types of iontophoresis units (Chayes-Seimon and 3M's Ionator) used metal, hand-held electrodes for the return. The patient held this in one hand while the brush tip was applied to the tooth. The hand-held elctrode is unfavorable because it can cause discomfort and the patient can vary the current by the amount of pressure applied or the amount of sweat present. In the Parkell's Desensitron system, the dentist completes the circuit by holding the hand on the patient's cheek. This is regarded, by the author, as the most unfavorable type of return electrode; a well attached, definite return pathway is preferred.

Figs. 25a and 25b Components of oral electrode (see also, Fig. 29).

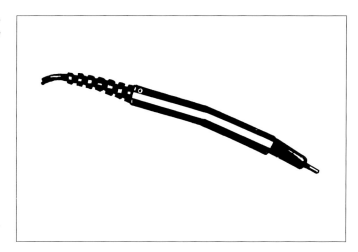

Fig. 25a Flexible oral electrode.

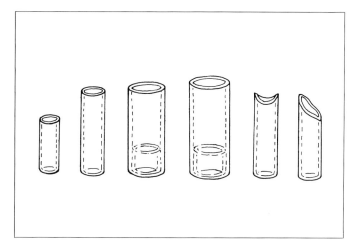

Fig. 25b Plastic tips for oral electrode.

Active Electrodes

The active electrodes described below are incorporated into the Dentelect Electro-Applicator System, Model C-2 (EAS).
Note: All electrodes and leads are color-coded so that positive or negative circuits can be easily distinguished during set-up and treatment. Red indicates positive and each red lead has a male snap attachment. Black is for negative and each black lead has a female snap attachment.

1. Oral electrodes: one red, one black
The *oral electrodes* are used for most dental applications. Figure 25a is a diagram of an *oral electrode*. It is insulated and flexible so as to be able to reach any area inside the mouth. One end contains a wire lead, attached to a male or female snap attachment, which fits the appropriate terminal of the Phoresor. At the other end there is an exposed metal tip which conducts current through an electrolyte drug soaking the cotton. A plastic *electrode tip* is fitted over the *oral electrode*, allowing

space for the cotton, and appropriately cut to adapt over and upon the teeth.

2. Plastic tips for oral electrode

The *plastic tips* which fit over the *oral electrode* are illustrated in Figure 25b. They are stuffed with cotton to receive the electrolyte solution. It is best to use only one piece of cotton in the tip. Inserting several pledgets could create air spaces between pledgets, thereby interfering with electrical conduction.

The tip selected depends upon the size and shape of the area to be treated. The end which touches the tooth is either straight-cut or can be contoured. Large tips are used for pre-injection topical or for treating lesions. *Plastic tips* which are contoured can be used to treat buccal or lingual surface of incisor, cuspid or molar teeth.

The *plastic tips* are very important for insulation. The rim of the tip is inserted below the gingival margins and this edge pushes the gingiva away from the lesion and prevents any current flow into gingiva. The complete assembly of an *oral electrode* and *electrode tips* is shown in Figure 31.

3. Clip electrodes: one red, one black

Clip electrodes are useful in the tray technique for treating multiple hypersensitivities simultaneously. (The tray technique is described in Chapter 13). The *clip electrode* is shown in Figure 26a. The alligator clip at one end attaches to an impression tray handle or onto a metal conductor. The other end of the clip electrode slips over a banana plug which is connected to a wire lead (GCL-1 or GCL-2) soldered to the appropriate snap attachment.

4. Brush electrodes: one red, one black

Brush electrodes are useful for treating lesions which are interproximal, at the gingival margin or subgingival, especially where a metal restoration exists near the lesion. A *brush electrode* is shown in Figure 26b. The brush fits over the *oral electrode*. Before attaching the brush to the *oral electrode*, the opening should be filled with the drug electrolyte (see Fig. 32). This gives an adequate supply of solution at the brush tip during the treatment. It should be noted that most of the previously marketed dental iontophoresors were supplied with only a brush electrode. The older configuration had two disadvantages (1) it is not suitable for many of the applications described in this monograph, and (2) the brush tended to loose its moisture during the iontophoresis. The new design of the brush (containing a reservoir) overcomes the latter problem. The author has found that the *brush electrode* has a few specific uses (see Chapter 13), but units which supply only brush electrodes lack the adaptability required of a modern iontophoresis system for dental practice.

5. Alternate accessories

The Dentelect ElectroApplicator, Model C-1 required banana plugs attached to oral and return leads, instead of the snap attachments adapted to the Phoresor. Snap attachments are more favorable, because there is no chance for improper connection.

6. Solutions

All drug solutions must be fresh and contain a minimum of contaminating ions.

A. Sodium nitrate (1%) was selected as the indifferent electrolyte because of its long history of use for pilocarpine iontophoresis. Although the author has found (unpublished observations) that during a 10 minute iontophoresis of sodium nitrate at 5 mA, the anodal solution can

Figs. 26a and 26b Clip and brush electrode (see also, Fig. 29).

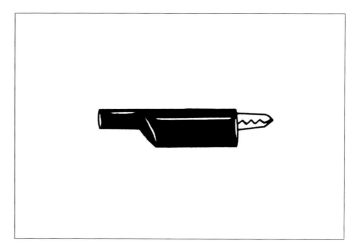

Fig. 26a   Clip electrode.

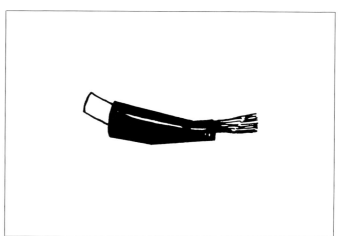

Fig. 26b   Brush electrode.

reach a pH of 1-2 and the cathodal, 13-14; such pronounced pH changes are not found in dental iontophoresis because fewer mA's are used. Thus tissue injury has almost never been observed from pH changes during dental use.

B. Ultrapure water (conductivity less than 3 μMHO). This solution is used to prepare and dilute drugs, thus avoiding any contaminating ions. De-ionized or distilled water is sufficient for this purpose and can be obtained from a pharmacy.

Drug Solutions

1. 2% sodium fluoride. This solution is used for the fluoride iontophoresis and is supplied with modern dental iontophoresors or can be obtained from a pharmacy.

Table 8 Polarity of Dental Drugs for Iontophoresis

Drug	Use	Active electrode		
		Polarity	Color	Snap
Lidocaine HCL (1-4%)	local anesthesia	+	red	male
Epinephrine HCL (1/10,000-1/50,000)	vasoconstrictor for local anesthesia	+	red	male
Fluoride (as 2% NaF)	desensitization of dentin	−	black	female
Solu-Medrol[R] (methyl-prednisolone sodium succinate)	anti-inflammatory for aphthous ulcer and lichen planus	−	black	female
Stoxil[R] (idoxuridine)	antiviral for herpes orolabialis	−	black	female

2. Local anesthetic-epinephrine. If the local anesthetic iontophoresis is routinely used for pre-injection topical anesthesia, it is best to mix the following solution, daily:

5 ml lidocaine 4% (obtain 5 ml ampules from the pharmacist)

1 ml epinephrine HC1 1/1000 (obtain 1 ml ampules from the pharmacist)

Mix 5 ml lidocaine with 0.5 ml of epinephrine. Dilute to 20 ml with ultrapure water. Final concentrations are lidocaine 1%, with adrenaline 1/40,000. The solution should be discarded when or if it shows brown coloration, and at the end of each day. Alternately, Xylocaine[R] 2% with 1/50,000 epinephrine may be used directly from a cartridge.

3. Solu-Medrol[R]. The pharmacist should prepare Solu-Medrol[R] as follows: 500 mg of drug is divided into 20 capsules containing 25 mg (±) 3 mg each. Just before use, 2 ml of water is added to the powder and the solution is ready for use. This solution should be mixed fresh daily. Any solution remaining at the end of a day should be discarded, because of instability.

4. Stoxil[R] Ophthalmic Solution, 0.1%. This is purchased from the pharmacy and kept refrigerated. This solution should last many months, according to its labelled shelf-life.

7. Polarity of drugs

Iontophoresis depends upon proper use of drug polarity. During development of iontophoresis for dental office use, one of the most frequent errors encountered by the author consisted of placement of drug at the wrong electrode. Because of this problem, EAS electrode leads are color coded. Table 8 is presented for reference so that the drug will be placed at the proper electrode.

8. Insulation:

The following materials are needed for insulation:

a. rubber dam and rubber dam accessories;

b. soft utility wax strips (Lactona[R] blue strips);

c. Masking tape; and

d. Copalite[R].

Techniques of insulation will be discussed under the specific protocols for desensitization of hypersensitive teeth (Chapter 13).

9. Impression materials are needed as follows:

a. alginate (conductive);

b. silastic or rubber impression material (non-conductive);

c. metal trays (locking type), assorted sizes; and

d. plastic trays, with holes, for partial impressions, assorted sizes.

The use of impression materials will be discussed under the specific protocols for the tray technique for treating multiple sensitivities (Chapter 13).

10. Saliva control is accomplished by the usual methods:

a. cotton rolls (when a rubber dam is not used);

b. aspirator;

c. probanthine, 15 mg, given 30-45 minutes pre-operatively for heavy salivators. A second capsule may be necessary if there is no effect (dry mouth) in 20-30 minutes.

11. Miscellaneous

Cotton pledgets, cotton rolls, disposable plastic dappen dishes (with calibrations from 1-30 ml), 1 and 5 cc syringes, 20 ga needles, gauze pads (2 × 2), and alcohol wipes.

Chapter 12

Operating Instructions for the ElectroApplicator System, Model C-2

Parts List — Dentelect Electrode-set™ by LPG adapted for the Phoresor[R] by Motion Control, Inc.

Cat. No.   Description

1. Power Supply,
   Phoresor[R] Model PM 600-2
2. Electrode Set
   DES-1   Dentelect Electrode Set™ by
             LPG (Complete)
3. Parts List for DES-1

Active Electrodes		No. per set
GOE-1	Red Oral Electrode	1
GOE-2	Black Oral Electrode	1
GCL-1	Red Lead for Clip	1
GCL-2	Black Lead for Clip	1
GCE-1	Red Clip Electrode	1
GCE-2	Black Clip Electrode	1
GBE-1[a]	Red Brush Electrode	1
GBE-2	Black Brush Electrode	1
Return Electrodes		
GRE-3	Female snap (−)	6
GRE-4	Male snap (+)	6

Tips for Oral Electrodes

GOE-3	Incisor Tip, one end straight-cut, one end contoured[b]	6
GOE-4	Cuspid Tip, one end straight-cut, one end contoured[b]	6
GOE-5	Molar Tip, straight-cut	2
GOE-6[c]	Molar Tip, contoured	2
GOE-7	Large Tips	4

4. Solutions: (Labelled for EXTERNAL USE ONLY)
   1% Sodium Nitrate
   2% Sodium Fluoride
   Ultrapure water (distilled or deionized)
5. Manual of Operating Instructions

[a]dropped; replaced by an extra GBE2
[b]both ends are now straight cut, contouring should be individualized by dentist or auxillary;
[c]contoured tips have been dropped (see footnote b.)

Description of ElectroApplicator System™

The Electroapplicator System™ consists of the Phoresor[R], Model PM 600-2, along with the Dentelect Electrode Set™ by LPG (Model DES-1). The Electrode Set contains all of the accessories necessary for safe and effective application of the iontophoretic technique in dental practice.

1. *Power supply*
Figure 27 is a reproduction of the Phoresor whose components are explained further.

A. is the treatment duration timer which is set for the number of minutes of treatment required. A reject occurs whenever the treatment timer is on zero and treatment is attempted. At the end of the procedure, the treatment duration timer terminates the current and a reject indicates that treatment is over.

B. is the dosage current display which gives a digital reading from 0.1 to 2.0 in mA to the nearest tenth.

C. is the current switch which contains an off-on mode and a rheostat for increasing voltage (and current).

D. is the reject panel containing two warning lights; the red flashing light (accompanied by an audible signal) indicates either 1) a faulty connection, 2) a faulty circuit, or 3) the end of treatment; the yellow light indicates that the battery is discharged.

E. is the output cable containing a negative terminal (F), a positive terminal (G), and an extension (H) for the positive terminal. (Note: the red dot on reverse side of H indicates (+) polarity.)

2. *Electrodes*
a. *Return electrode*
The *return electrodes* (GRE-3 and GRE-4) supplied with the ElectroApplicator System™ are similar to band-aids, and have male(+) or female(−) snaps. The snaps are attached to the appropriate terminal of the *output cable*. Pads are contained over the conductive snaps which protect the skin from the metal and are used to hold the drug. The return electrodes are disposable for convenience in handling. Figure 28 shows the steps in application of the return electrode to the patient.

b. *Active electrodes*
1) *Oral electrodes* (Fig. 29a)
Two *oral electrodes* are provided, one red (GOE-1) and one black (GOE-2). Each electrode is an insulated flexible probe and a wire lead of the same color. The flexibility makes it possible to bend the electrode to reach any area in the oral cavity. The opposite end of each lead has a snap attachment to connect the electrode to the appropriate terminal of the *Phoresor output cable*. The end of each probe has exposed metal through which current is conducted. *Plastic electrode tips* (GOE-3, 4, 5, and 7) are provided to fit over the end of the *oral electrode*. *Brush electrodes* (GBE-1 and GBE-2) also fit over the *oral electrodes*.

2) *Electrode tips* (Fig. 29b)
The *electrode tips* are plastic tubes which fit over the end of the *oral electrode*. Tips are supplied in six configurations: 1) incisor size (GOE-3) is straight-cut at one end and contoured-cut at the other; 2) cuspid size (GOE-4) fits cuspids and bicuspids, and also is straight-cut at one end and contoured-cut at the other; 3) small molar size (GOE-5) is straight-cut; 4) small molar size (GOE-6) is contoured-cut; and 5)

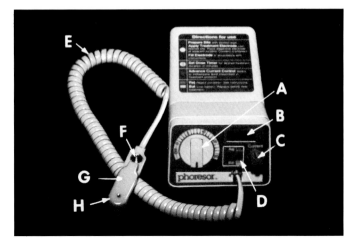

Fig. 27 Phoresor™ model PM-2 as specified for dental iontophoresis: a) treatment duration timer, b) dosage current display, c) current switch, d) reject panel, e) output cable, f) negative terminal, g) positive terminal, h) extension.

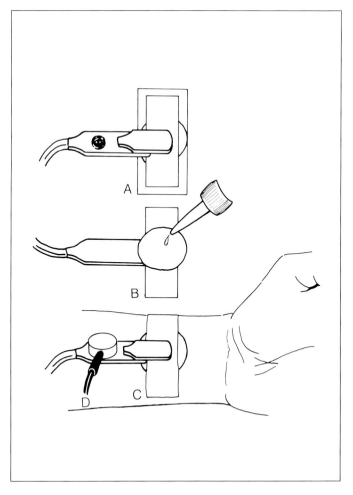

Fig. 28 Application and connection of return electrode: a) Return electrode connected to positive terminal of *output cable;* b) Soaking the pad with 1% sodium nitrate; c) Applied to skin; d) Active electrode.

Connection of return electrode:
1. Swab the volar surface of the forearm with alcohol and allow to dry.
2. Select a male return electrode (GRE-4) for application of a negative drug such as fluoride while a female (GRE-3) return electrode is selected for application of a positive drug.
3. Snap the return electrode into the appropriate terminal (A).
4. Apply the indifferent electrolyte, sodium nitrate (1%) to the pad. Shake off any excess fluid so that the adhesive on the tape does not become wet.
5. Attach to arm stretching the tape slightly so that the pad is flat against the skin.

Summary and Uses of Active Electrodes

Electrodes	Uses

A. Oral Electrode (GOE-1 and GOE-2)

Use with Plastic Tips (B) or Brush Electrode (C)
1. Desensitize cervical area
2. Desensitize crown preparation
3. Preinjection topical
4. Treatment of a lesion

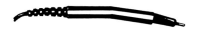

B. Plastic Tips (GOE-3, 4, 5, 7)

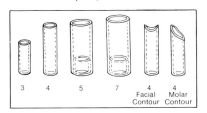

Tips for Oral Electrode (GOE-1 or GOE-2)
1. Desensitize cervical area
2. Desensitize crown preparation
3. Preinjection topical anesthesia
4. Treatment of a lesion

C. Brush Electrode (GBE-1 and GBE-2)

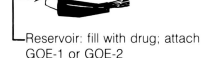

Reservoir: fill with drug; attach GOE-1 or GOE-2

Connect Brush to GOE-1 or GOE-2
1. Desensitize exposed dentin at or below gingival margin
2. Desensitize an interproximal area
3. Desensitize surface of last molar

D. Clip Electrode (GCE-1 and GCE-2)

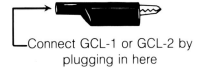

Connect GCL-1 or GCL-2 by plugging in here

1. Clip to metal tray handle to densensitize a quadrant
2. Clip to metal wire inserted into rubber base impression to desensitize several crown preparations
3. Clip to GTA trays for mucosal anesthesia

Figure 29

large, lesion size (GOE-7) is straight-cut. (Note: GOE-6 and GOE-8, as well as contours on GOE-3 and GOE-4 have been omitted from DES-1, see footnotes page 99). Straight-cup tips are used to fit lesions which are not on curving surfaces. Contoured tips will fit over cavity and crown preparations, adapting to the gingival margin, and are also useful to adapt to curved facial and lingual surfaces of teeth. Contouring can be easily accomplished by the operator.

3) *Brush electrodes* (Fig. 29c)
Two black brush electrodes (GBE-2) are provided. (Note: GBE-1 red brush electrode has been omitted from DES-1 but can be obtained by special order.) The brush electrode consists of an insulator over the metal brush which is fitted with a plastic tip; the latter engages the end of the oral electrode. Brush electrodes are useful for treating interproximal, gingival-marginal or subgingival lesions, especially when metal restorations are near the lesion. Prior to use, the plastic tube and the metal part of the brush are filled with electrolyte, which acts as a reservoir and conducts current from oral electrode to the metal part of brush. The reservoir feature is an improvement over other currently marketed products because the brush tip does not dry out when a reservoir is present.

4) *Clip electrodes and clip electrode leads* (Fig. 29d)
Two *clip electrodes* are provided, 1 red (GCE-1) and 1 black (GCE-2). Each clip electrode consists of an insulated alligator clip which is used for attachment to an impression tray handle or a metal conductor. GCE-1 fits onto GCL-1 and GCE-2 fits onto GCL-2.

5) *Electrode leads for clip electrodes*

Two color-coded *electrode leads* for *clip electrodes* GCL-1 and GCL-2 are provided, 1 red (GCL-1) and 1 black (GCL-2). Each *lead* has a banana-jack at one end and a snap attachment at the other. The banana-jack plugs into the appropriate *clip electrode* while the snap attachment is secured to the appropriate *terminal* of the *output cable*. (Note: GCL-1 was formerly GRE-1 and GCL-2 was formerly GRE-2).

3. *Solutions*
Powders and bottles are supplied with the ElectroApplicator System™ so that the following solutions can be made:
   2% sodium fluoride (NaF)
   1% sodium nitrate (NaNO$_3$)
   ultrapure water (distilled or de-ionized water).
Follow directions supplied with the packets for making solutions.

General Operating Instruction for Electroapplicator System™

1. Read instruction manual completely, prior to using instrument.
2. Select the proper drug for the condition to be treated (see Table 8). Use only fresh, pure drugs of proper concentration.
3. Make sure the battery of the Phoresor™ power supply is not discharged. If the battery is low, a yellow signal on the face of the unit will appear after the unit is turned on. If so, replace with a new 9V alkaline transistor battery. Prior to use, the *current switch* should be in the *off* position.
4. Select the proper polarity for the drug to be used (see Table 8). This is opposite in polarity to the *return electrode*. Note: the *return electrode* may establish the polarity of the system; for

example, in desensitization of sensitive teeth, the negative drug fluoride is to be applied, so the male *return electrode* is selected for connection to the *positive terminal* of the *power supply*.

5. As shown in Figs. 28 a, b and c, the *return electrode* (GRE-3, female or GRE-4, male) is applied to the skin of the forearm, and the *return electrode* snap attached to the *terminal* of the Phoresor. The appropriate *return electrode* is first attached to the correct *terminal* of the Phoresor (Fig. 28a). The male *return electrode* is positive and is snapped into the *positive terminal* of the Phoresor *output cable* when a negative drug is to be used at the *active electrode*. The female *return electrode* is negative and attached to the male snap of the Phoresor *output cable* when positive drugs are administered at the *active electrode*. After attachment, the *return electrode* backing is removed and about 1 cc of 1% sodium nitrate solution is applied to the paper support (Fig. 28b) until soaked. The skin of forearm is swabbed with alcohol and the *return electrode* is taped to the volar surface of patient's forearm (Fig. 28c). The tape is stretched gently to help keep the pad flat against the skin. Another piece of tape (adhesive) may be placed against the electrode assembly to help secure the *return electrode*. Additional sodium nitrate may be added to the electrode pad to keep it saturated; excess solution should be wiped from the arm.

6. Select the appropriate active electrode (*oral electrode*, GOE-1 or GOE-2), *brush electrode* (GBE-1 or 2) or *clip electrode* (GCE-1 or 2), depending upon the area to be treated. The brush is used for areas which are difficult to reach or when difficulty is ex-

perienced in obtaining insulation. The *clip electrodes* are used for tray techniques. Specific instructions for use of each of these electrode configurations are included under the protocols for desensitization (Chapter 13). For example, when the negatively charged drug, sodium fluoride is to be applied, the black GOE-2 is selected and connected to the *negative terminal* of the power supply cord. A summary of active electrodes with appropriate connections and uses, was made above (Fig. 29 a). After selecting the oral electrode, a plastic tip (Fig. 29b), of appropriate type and size to fit the area of treatment, is chosen.

7. Apply drug to the appropriate *electrode tip* according to instructions for the specific condition to be treated. Apply the active electrode to the area of treatment. When the *electrode tips* are used, it is important that the cotton saturated with the drug comes in contact with entire area of tissue being treated. It is important that the area under treatment be kept moist during the treatment, and, when treating teeth, the soft tissues must be insulated. The plastic *electrode tip* will adequately insulate the gingiva; wax, masking tape or Copalite (two coats) is used to insulate metal restorations. For the tray technique, a rubber dam is used to insulate the gingiva and the tray; or, the tray is made nonconductive by using rubber base impressions in acrylic trays.

8. Turn *treatment duration timer* past 5 minutes: Turn *current switch* to *on*. (A single beep signals that the unit is on.) Slowly turn *current switch* clockwise to increase the current to the desired level and note this on the digital display. The treatment mA level is determined by the patient's comfort or by

preset limits, whichever is less. For preset limits, see instructions for the specific techniques, which are discussed further in Chapter 13-16 for each specific protocol.

9. Set the *treatment duration timer* to the desired number of minutes for the treatment. The current will be maintained constant and be turned off by the *timer* at the end of the period.

10. If treatment must be stopped for any reason, note the time of treatment completed, turn *current switch* to *off,* and correct any problems. Then, resume treatment by repeating steps 8 and 9; however, *timer* is reset to administer only the uncompleted treatment. For example, if the total treatment time was 2 minutes, and one minute of treatment was uncompleted, set *timer* to one minute after reconnection of the patient.

11. When the treatment is completed, turn the *current switch* to the *off* position and remove the electrodes from the patient.

Chapter 13

Instructions: Desensitization of Hypersensitive Dentin

General Summary

1. Drug—2% NaF for most procedures (exception: 1% NaF is used when alginate is the electrode material (see Tray Techniques).
2. Drug polarity is negative—use black *electrodes*.
3. *Return electrode* is positive—use GRE-4 (Male (+) snap). Saturate pad with $NaNO_3$.
4. Maximum safe current level (mA)
   Single tooth—0.5 mA or at threshold level.
   Tray technique—0.5 mA per tooth, up to 2 mA maximum, or at patient's threshold level, whichever is less.
   Maximum safe current dosage—1.0 mA-min per tooth.
5. *Active electrode* selection
   a. For single tooth: either GOE-2 with appropriate *plastic tip* (GOE-3, 4, 5, or 7) or GOE-2 with *brush tip* (GBE-2).
   b. For tray technique, (GCE-2 with GCL-2) *clip electrode*
6. *Usual* steps for desensitization of a single hypersensitive tooth. Assume treatment is on facial of a cuspid.
   a. Apply *oral electrode* (GOE-2) to the Phoresor *output cable*.
   b. Assemble active *electrode tip* (GOE-4) and fill with cotton.
   c. Apply NaF to cotton in GOE-4.
   *d. Apply return electrode (GRE-4, male) to Phoresor *output cable*.
   e. Apply $NaNO_3$ to *return electrode*.
   f. Apply *return electrode* to skin of forearm.
   g. Turn *timer* to past 5 min.
   h. Apply *oral electrode* to tooth completing the circuit.
   i. Turn *current switch* on and increase gradually to 0.5 mA.
   j. Return *timer* to 2 minutes.
   k. At end of procedure, remove electrodes and test with air.

Diagnosis: Location and Severity of Dentinal Lesions

This is a most important part of your treatment plan. The subject of diagnosis was covered above in Chapter 8, but a few additional comments will serve to remind the reader of some practical aspects of diagnosis.

You should accurately chart each sensitive area, determining if the lesion is treatable by iontophoresis (consider caries, irreversible pulpitis and cracked tooth as non-treatable by iontophoresis or better treated by other methods). An example of a chart for recording sensi-

*Steps d, e, and f can precede a, b, and c.

tivity was included above (Fig. 18). A copy of this or another record-keeping chart should be included with the patient's folder.

In order to diagnose hypersensitive teeth, use the following format:

1. *Select stimulus for testing:*
   a. Cold air blast (one second); this is usually used by the author;
   b. Ice water (0.2 ml); directed at each tooth area; this distinguishes between exposed dentin sensitivity and thermal shocks from dentin under restorations;
   c. Explorer touch; carry the explorer lightly, but firmly, across each suspected surface; or
   d. Grapefruit juice, for acrid foods.

Note: In extreme cases of multiple, intolerable sensitivities, the pretreatment diagnosis may be eliminated (see Step 4).

2. *Perform the test and chart sensitive areas:*

While directing cold stimulus at a particular area of a tooth, you must insulate the adjacent areas with your fingers or by some other method. This is especially important for distinguishing between buccofacial and interproximal sensitivity.

Train the patient to rate the sensitivity as follows:

0 = normal, 1 = mild discomfort, 2 = moderate, 3 = severe but transient, 4 = intolerable, severe and lasting.

3. *Decide on the best method of treating the sensitive areas and present your treatment plan to the patient.*
   a. For a single tooth you may wish to perform the fluoride iontophoresis

immediately so as to complete diagnosis and treatment in one appointment.
   b. For multiple scattered hypersensitive teeth, you may wish to divide the work into several appointments, treating 2-4 (or more) teeth per appointment.
   c. For multiple hypersensitivities concentrated in quadrants or arch segments, you may wish to treat each arch segment (or an entire arch) with a tray technique. This is especially useful for postperiodontal surgery patients with a great amount of interproximal sensitivity. The alginate tray technique is described later in this chapter.
   d. For crown preparations or extensive cavity preparations, the fluoride iontophoresis should be done when extensive dentin is exposed. Prepared teeth can be treated either individually, when there are one or two teeth needing treatment, or in arch segments, when 3 or more teeth require treatment. The use of the rubber base impression as the electrode is helpful for desensitizing 3 or more crown preparations or bridge abutments.

4. *Post-treatment diagnosis:*

The pretreatment diagnostic procedures are repeated, using the same stimulus and the results recorded on the same chart. If retreatments are needed, additional appointments are scheduled at one week intervals.

An additional post-treatment diagnostic procedure is to test reaction to a rinse with tap water, ice water, or grapefruit juice (if the problem is acrid foods). This test is useful if the patient has multiple sensitivities and cannot tolerate the pretreatment diagnostic procedures.

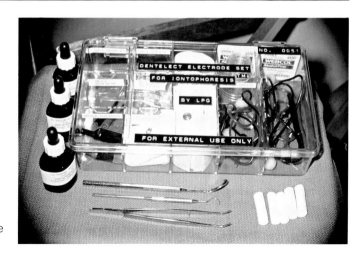

Fig. 30   Tray set-up for fluoride iontophoresis.

Spot Desensitization of a Single Tooth Using a Plastic Tip

1. Materials needed (Fig. 30).
    Phoresor
    2% NaF
    GRE-4, *return electrode*
    1% $NaNO_3$
    GOE-2, *active electrode*
    Plastic tip (GOE-3, 4, 5) Selection of tip depends on tooth size. Tips are contoured according to surface under treatment.
    Cotton batting
2. Maximum safe current and current dosage.
    0.5 mA
    1.0 mA-min
3. *Active electrode* assembly (Fig. 31).
    The GOE-2 is snapped into the appropriate *terminal* of the *Phoresor output* and bent to an appropriate angle for convenience of application. The GOE-tip is placed over end of GOE-2. One wisp of cotton is obtained from the batting (or a cotton roll) so that the tip is slightly overfilled. The cotton is then soaked with 2% NaF solution assuring that the solution reaches the metal of the GOE-2. For smaller teeth use the GOE-3, for medium teeth the GOE-4, and for larger teeth, the GOE-5. However, many molars can be treated with GOE-4, using it uncut or contoured as shown in Figure 29. Also *plastic tips* are used over crown preparations, with contoured-ends adapting to facial surface or cotton wisps stuffed around the preparation.
4. Application of return (skin) electrode (Fig. 28)
    The GRE-4 is snapped into the *positive terminal* of the *output cable*. A piece of adhesive tape may be placed over the assembled *output cable* to hold it flat against the arm.
5. Insulation.
    a. The plastic tips will often provide sufficient insulation for the gingiva if properly placed on the tooth. Therefore, cotton rolls can be used to wall off the area and no rubber dam is needed. Contoured tips are especially useful for adapting to the gingiva. A blanching of the gingiva during treatment indicates that a seal is obtained. The tips should be well

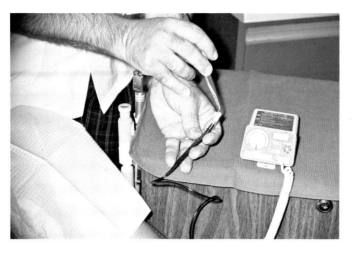

Figs. 31a, 31b and 31c Active electrode assembly and use.

Fig. 31a Oral electrode assembly.

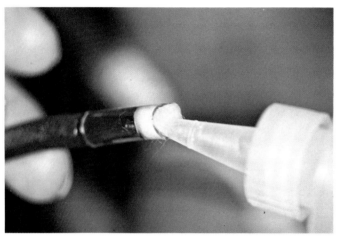

Fig. 31b Close-up of solution application to tip.

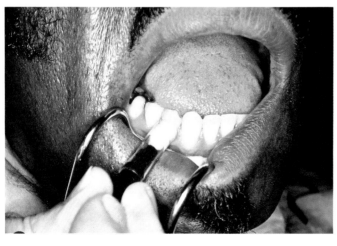

Fig. 31c Close-up of treatment and use. Note how Plastic Tip fits facial surface and seals the gingiva, providing insulation.

adapted to the tooth with cotton touching the entire lesion and enough pressure applied to blanch the gingiva during the whole procedure.

b. If it is determined that a rubber dam is desirable, it is placed over the teeth to be treated. Suction should be used to keep the field dry if the patient is a heavy salivator.

c. Metallic restorations which could be contacted by the electrode are carefully covered with either soft blue utility wax (Lactona brand), masking tape or 2 coats of Copalite[R] Be careful not to cover the exposed dentin lesion.

6. Clean and dry the teeth.

Pledgets of cotton or gauze pads are used to wipe the surface to be treated. This removes the plaque; thus, a prophy is not required. Air is avoided for the drying, but may be used gently.

7. Set the *treatment duration timer* to past 5 minutes.

8. Connect active electrode to lesion (Fig. 31).

Slowly turn up the *current switch* until the patient feels a slight sensation in the tooth or in the arm. Adjust the current downward to eliminate any uncomfortable sensation.

9. *Maximum current.*

Do not exceed 0.5 mA when treating a single tooth.

10. *Maximum current dosage.*

Do not exceed 1.0 mA-min when treating a single tooth. Use the following schedule as a guide to obtain 1mA-min:

0.5 mA—2 min (the usual settings for most treatments)
0.4 mA—3 min
0.3 mA—4 min
0.2 mA—5 min

Set the *timer* to appropriate number of minutes. Current duration must be increased if cotton contacts gingiva during the treatment. Double current duration if electrode is $1/2$ on gingiva and $1/2$ on tooth.

11. Test with air or 0.2 ml ice-water per tooth.

If relief is not complete, the procedure may be repeated once or twice, at weekly intervals. Be sure to warn the patient, before starting that three treatments may be needed.

Desensitization of a Tooth Using a Brush Electrode

1. Materials needed
   2% NaF
   GRE-4, return electrode
   1% $NaNO_3$
   GOE-2, oral electrode with GBE-2, brush electrode (Fig. 29c).

2. Maximum safe current.

For isolated tooth–0.5 mA (*Note:* Increase up to 1.0 mA when contacting gingiva or for interproximal sensitivity when touching two teeth).

1.0 mA-min per tooth (*Note:* Increase to 2.0 mA-min per tooth when touching gingiva).

3. *Active electrode* assembly (Figs. 32 a, b, and c)

The GOE-2 is snapped into the appropriate terminal of the *Phoresor output cable* and bent to an appropriate angle for convenience of application. The GBE-2 is filled with 2% NaF from the reservoir side (Fig. 32a) and placed over GOE-2 (Fig. 32b).

4. Application of return (skin) electrode (Fig. 28)

The GRE-4 is snapped into the *positive terminal* of the *output cable*. A piece of adhesive tape may be placed over the *output cable* to hold it flat against the arm.

5. Insulation

The area to be treated is insulated, to whatever extent is possible. (However, the brush technique is usually used because

111

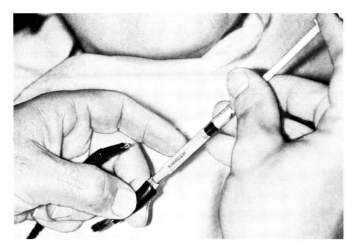

Figs. 32a, 32b, 32c   Assembly of brush electrode.

Fig. 32a   Filling the reservoir.

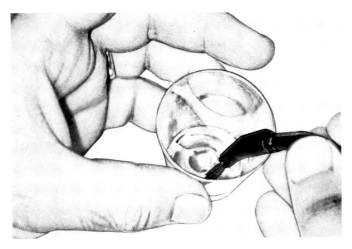

Fig. 32b   Wetting bristles of assembled electrode.

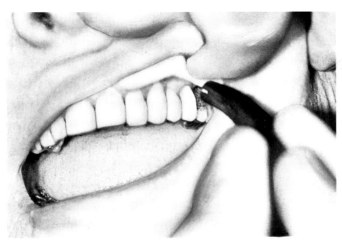

Fig. 32c   Application to the sensitive area.

complete insulation cannot be obtained.) Follow any steps which are considered useful. The amount of insulation obtained affects the current and current-duration in the brush technique.

6. Clean and dry the teeth

Pledgets of cotton or gauze pads are used to wipe the surface to be treated. This removes the plaque; thus, a prophy is not required. Air is avoided for drying, but may be used gently.

7. Turn *timer* to on.

Set the *treatment duration timer* to past 5 min

8. Apply *brush* to lesion.

Soak the bristles of the *brush electrode* in 2% NaF and apply to lesion (Fig. 32c); slowly turn up the *current switch* until the patient feels a slight sensation in the tooth or in the arm. Adjust the current downward to eliminate any uncomfortable sensation.

9. Current maximum

If the brush is totally on an insulated single tooth, do not exceed 0.5 mA. If loss is occurring through the gingiva, the current may be increased to 1.0 mA.

10. Maximum current dosage

Do not exceed 1.0 mA-min if the brush is on an insulated tooth. If loss of current into gingiva is occurring, double treatment time or increase current rate to obtain twice as much current-dosage. If two teeth are being treated, another multiple of two is used. (For example, 1.0 mA for 4 min.) Use the following schedule for brush electrode treatment:

a. Single insulated tooth—1.0 mA-min (0.5 mA for 2 min)

b. Single tooth with loss of current through gingiva—2.0 mA-min

> 0.5 mA for 4 min
> 0.7 mA for 3 min
> 1.0 mA for 2 min

c. Interproximal, two teeth with rubber dam insulation—1.0 mA-min/tooth or 2.0 mA-min

d. Interproximal, two teeth with loss of current through gingiva—2.0 mA-min/tooth

> 0.5 mA for 8 min
> 0.7 mA for 6 min
> 1.0 mA for 4 min
> 1.4 mA for 3 min

Set the *timer* to appropriate number of minutes as described in schedule above.

11. Test with air or 0.2 ml ice-water per tooth

If relief is not complete, the procedure may be repeated once or twice at *weekly* intervals.

Desensitization of a Segment of an Arch or an Entire Arch (the *Tray Technique*)

1. Drug—1% sodium fluoride (Note: 1% NaF is used instead of 2% because the latter causes deterioration of the alginate).

2. Active electrode—black *clip electrode* (GCE-2) attached to GCL-2.

3. Application of *return electrode* (GRE-4) (Fig. 28).

4. Preparation of active electrode. Take an impression of the arch in a metal tray using alginate. Cut out alginate areas of arch which will *not* be treated, but leave impressions of all teeth to be treated intact (Fig. 33a). Wrap impression in a wet towel (tap water).

5. Insulation. Place a full size (6″ × 6″) piece of rubber dam over the teeth to be treated, isolating all teeth under treatment (Fig. 33b). Apply either masking tape, pieces of soft utility wax or two coats of Copalite[R] over any metal restorations in the field under treatment.

6. Clean and dry teeth by wiping with gauze and cotton and using suction to keep treatment area saliva-free.

Figs. 33a through 33g Alginate tray technique for treating multiple hypersensitivities.

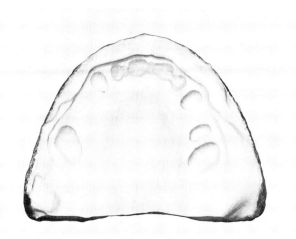

Fig. 33a Trimmed alginate impression.

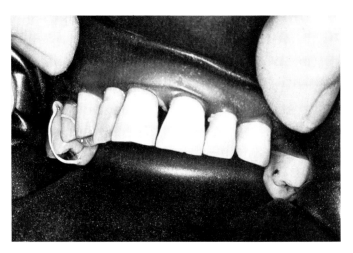

Fig. 33b Application of rubber dam.

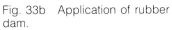

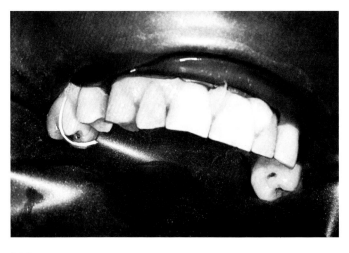

Fig. 33c Application of cotton between teeth.

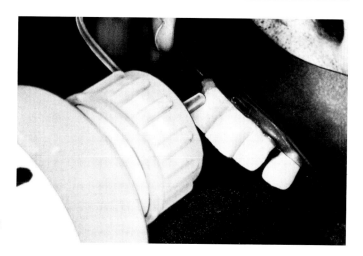

Fig. 33d Soaking teeth and cotton with NaF solution.

7. Turn *Phoresor treatment duration timer* to past 10 min.
8. Prepare teeth for tray electrode insertion: 1) stuff cotton between teeth where there is interproximal sensitivity (Fig. 33c); 2) apply sodium fluoride to teeth and cotton (Fig. 33d) and into impression (Fig. 33e); and 3) insert impression over teeth, wrapping it completely with the rubber dam (Fig. 33f) to insulate metal tray from the oral soft tissues. Secure the clip electrode onto the tray handle (Fig. 33g).
9. Slowly turn up the *current switch* until the patient feels a tickling sensation either in teeth or arm. Adjust current downward to eliminate any uncomfortable sensation. Up to 2.0 mA can be used.
10. Current duration—1.0 mA min. per tooth. This procedure is usually performed at 1.0 mA, then the *timer* is set for a number of minutes equal to the number of teeth under treatment. (Example: 6 teeth—use 6.0 mA-min or six minutes at 1.0 mA.) If current level is set higher, divide mA into mA-min to calculate minutes of treatment.
11. Test with air or 0.2 ml ice water per tooth. If relief is only partial, the procedure may be repeated once or twice, at weekly intervals, or spot desensitization may be performed later.

The alginate tray procedure is effective for cases of hypersensitivity after periodontal surgery. Cotton should be liberally applied between teeth after placement of rubber dam. This procedure may also be useful for topical fluoride treatment, since the impression keeps the fluoride in close contact with the enamel while the current aids delivery of fluoride. This should be the best method of quickly introducing fluoride into dentin; some preliminary results from our laboratories indicate increased fluoride uptake and increased acid resistance of both enamel and dentin after fluoride iontophoresis, compared to topical application.

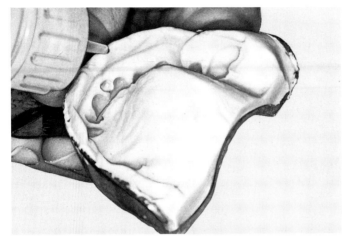

Fig. 33e Loading impression with NaF solution.

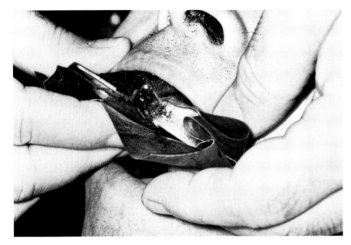

Fig. 33f Reinsertion of impression.

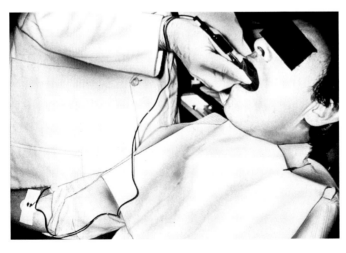

Fig. 33g Complete set-up for fluoride iontophoresis.

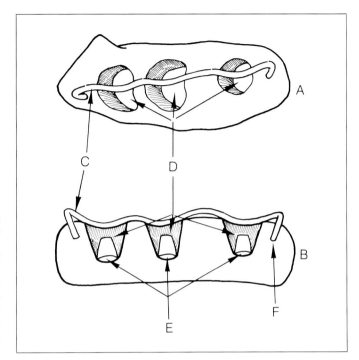

Fig. 34 Schematic showing preparation of rubber base impression for tray technique: a) top view: three-dimension occlusal view, b) side view: cross-sectional view, c) wire: to receive clip electrode, d) rubber removed: Fill space with cotton to hold electrolyte, e) gingival margins: Keep intact, f) holes for insertion of wires.

Desensitization of Multiple Crown Preps (modification of *the Tray Technique*)

Since a rubber base impression is usually available, a modification of the Tray Technique is used. All steps are the same as described above except for steps 4 and 5. 1-3. (see *the Tray Technique* page 113)
4. Preparation of active electrode. The rubber base impression, with the following modification, is used as the active electrode (Fig. 34). The impression material around the abutments is removed with a large round bur working from the occlusal side; the gingival margins must be carefully preserved. Two holes are made in the plastic on the occlusal side of the tray so that a piece of wire can be inserted into the holes over the abutment teeth.

5. Insulation. By preserving the gingival margins, no further insulation is needed since rubber contacts the soft tissues. Any metallic restorations are insulated with Copalite[R] or wax. The modified impression is inserted and cotton is packed around the teeth so that the cotton touches all of the dentin and the metal wire; the cotton is saturated with 2% NaF (Fig. 34).
6-11 (see the *Tray Technique,* pages 113-115)
Note: Some of the procedures in step 8, p. 115 were accomplished in steps 4 and 5.)

Figures 35 a, b, c, d, e, f show the steps in rubber base *tray desensitization* of multiple bridge abutments. Because of the importance of this *tray technique* in dentin desensitization of abutments or crown preparations, the case report for the patient illustrated in Fig. 35 will be presented. Mrs. S. W. was a 47-year-old, healthy female having had orthognathic surgery and crown preparations on 16 teeth. Two teeth (#9, #25) were devital. During crown preparation, all vital cut teeth of both arches (Fig. 35a) became extremely sensitive and there was much discomfort to thermal changes, even with the temporary crowns in place. One other source of discomfort was exercising, which may have caused pain due to hyperemia related to nerve damage during orthognathic surgery. The prepared teeth were not rated prior to iontophoresis treatment because the slightest flow of air on any vital tooth caused excruciating discomfort. In such cases, we recommend fluoride iontophoresis on all the crown preparations by a *tray technique* using the rubber base impressions to carry the fluoride. When rubber base impressions are available, it is favorable to prepare the trays as the electrode carrier by the method described below; the gingival and soft tissue adaptation of the rubber provides excellent insulation without the need for a rubber dam.

The impressions (Fig. 35b) were prepared as follows:

1. A small round bur was used to make openings through the rubber and acrylic of each impression, starting from the tissue side.
2. With the openings as guides, a large acrylic bur was used to further open the areas of the impression around each crown, working from the occlusal side. It is important to leave the gingival margin intact for the purpose of insulation.
3. The impressions were tried in the mouth to determine if any more rubber should be removed. Ideally, all of the dentin of the preparation should be exposed, when the impression is in place, but the gingival margins should be sealed.
4. A piece of 22 gauge wire was adapted over the occlusal surface and held in place on the impression by two right angle bends, which fitted into the acrylic of the impression distal to the last preparations. This wire was used to carry the current into the exposed dentin. Figure 35c demonstrates the completed maxillary impression inserted into the mouth.
5. Cotton wisps were tucked around each preparation so as to completely surround each tooth (Fig. 35d). Any metal restorations must be insulated with wax (for example, tooth #9, a non-vital tooth which had a post and coping). Figure 35d also shows that tooth #13 had not yet been surrounded with cotton.
6. The cotton around all teeth was soaked with 2% NaF (Fig. 35e) and the wire inserted into place (see step 4). Figure 35f demonstrates the completed tray electrode, in place, with the *alligator clip* (GCE-2) attached to the wire. It may be necessary to place additional cotton between the wire and some preparations; all preparations must make contact through wet cotton to the wire. Aspiration was used to remove excess fluoride solution and to prevent saliva contamination.
7. The *clip electrode lead* (GCL-2) and clip electrode (GCE-2) were connected to the negative terminal of the Phoresor. The *return electrode,* soaked with 2% sodium nitrate, was connected to the skin of the forearm (Fig. 35g).
8. Current was passed through the wire and through the cotton into the dentin, using 1.0 mA-min per tooth.
9. When the audible signal sounded,

Figs. 35a through 35g Rubber base tray technique for treating multiple crown preparations.

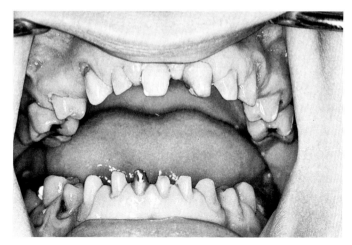

Fig. 35a Patient with multiple crown preparations.

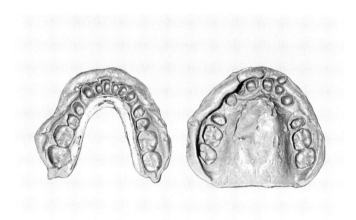

Fig. 35b Rubber dam impressions.

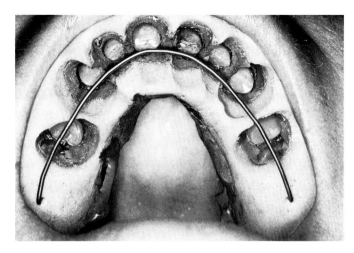

Fig. 35c Upper impression inserted over teeth. (Note wire placement.)

119

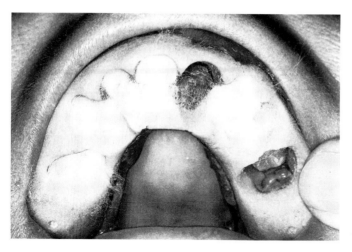

Fig. 35d Insertion of cotton around preparations. (Note wax insulation over metallic coping in devital tooth #9.)

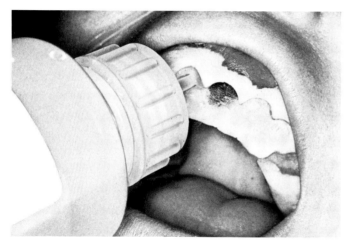

Fig. 35e Application of NaF to cotton.

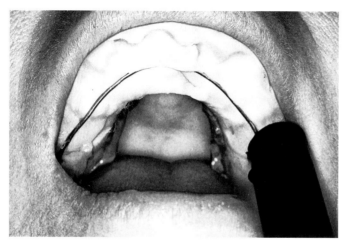

Fig. 35f Application of clip electrode to wire (lower right).

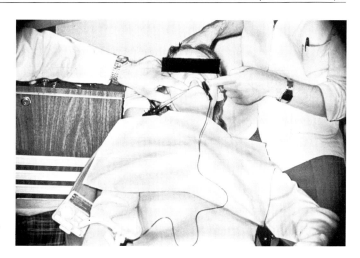

Fig. 35g Complete set-up for iontophoresis.

treatment was complete and the tray was removed.

10. The impression is saved in case a second treatment is needed. Also, if a few areas remain sensitive, spot desensitization can be performed at a later appointment.

The results for this patient (and many others performed by the author and other dentists) were very satisfactory. The patient felt mild to moderate discomfort from the air blasts immediately after the treatment. She was able to tolerate air flow and tap water in her mouth. Only two teeth required further spot desensitization. Further try-ins crown and cementation were performed without use of anesthesia. Six weeks after cementation, the patient still had discomfort when exercising, but there was no evidence of thermal sensitivity. (We believe the exercise discomfort was related to nerve damage due to orthognathic surgery).

Chapter 14

Instructions for Use in Surface Local Anesthesia

(Preinjection topical or for extraction of loose deciduous teeth or for gingival therapy.)

Summary

1. Drugs—use either:
   a. 2% Lidocaine HCl with 1/50,000 epinephrine (Xylocaine^R green carpules); or
   b. 4% Lidocaine—5 ml ampule and 1/1000 epinephrine HCl-1 ml ampule; open the ampules and add 0.5 ml epinephrine to 5 ml of lidocaine in a dappen dish, dilute to 20 ml with ultrapure water. Mix this solution fresh daily.

Drug polarity is positive.

2. Return electrode—negative

Use 1% sodium nitrate as the indifferent electrolyte.

3. Maximum current: 1.0 mA for GOE Tips; 2.0 mA for GTA trays or large areas.

4. Active electrode selection

Oral electrode with straight cut *plastic tip* for preinjection topical.

GTA-*trays* for deciduous tooth extraction or for gingival therapy.

Preinjection Topical

1. Select drug; Xylocaine^R green cartridge solution (a, above) or 1% lidocaine with 1/40,000 epinephrine (step b, above).
2. Active electrode selection. Use red *oral electrode* (GOE-1) with straight-cut, large *electrode tip* (GOE-5 or 7).
3. Assemble and place female *return* (skin) *electrode* (Fig. 28). Snap into the negative lead of the *output cable*.
4. Preparation of active electrode

The red *oral electrode* is snapped into the *positive* (red) *terminal* of the *output cable*. Bend flexible *oral electrode* to desired angle for ease of application. Insert an electrode *tip* and fill with cotton, leaving it overfilled by 2–3 mm. Apply lidocaine-epinephrine solution to the *tip,* being certain that the saturated cotton touches the metal.

5. The *treatment duration timer* is turned to 10 minutes.
6. Connect active electrode to the area to be anesthetized; turn on *current switch,* increasing it until the patient feels a tickling sensation in the mucosa or in the arm. Adjust current downward to eliminate any uncomfortable sensation.
7. Current maximum: Do not exceed 1.0 mA or patient threshold.
8. Current duration: Set *treatment duration timer* for 2 to 4 minutes (2.0 mA-min are needed). After current stops, wait for 2 minutes for anesthesia to become complete.

Note: Insulate any metal restoration which might touch cotton tip.

Extraction of Loose Deciduous Teeth or Gingival Therapy (gingival curettage or other treatment of gingiva)

1. Description of GTA-*trays* for mucosal anesthesia. (*Note:* GTA trays are supplied separately; they are not part of the EAS).
    a. There are *five trays* in the GTA series (Fig. 36); each *tray* is intended to be used in a different area of the mouth.
    b. *Labels* are included with each *tray;* attach labels to your DES organizer tray; so that GTA-*trays* are identified.
    c. Design and Selection of GTA Trays.
    GTA-*1* is an anterior tray, useful for gingival and mucosal anesthesia around 1 or 2 teeth. GTA-1 is used for extraction of loose deciduous teeth, for gingival curettage or for other treatment of the gingiva. GTA-1 is shown in cross-sectional view in Figure 36 I, and in perspective view in Figure 36 IV (upper left).
    GTA-*2* is a small posterior tray useful for gingival and mucosal anesthesia around 2 or 3 teeth. GTA-2 is used for extraction of loose deciduous teeth, for gingival curettage or other operations on the gingiva. GTA-2 is shown in cross-sectional view in Figure 36 I, and in perspective view in Figure 36 IV (upper middle).
    GTA-*3* is a large posterior tray useful for gingival and mucosal anesthesia around 3 or 4 teeth. GTA-3 is used for gingival curettage or other operations on the gingiva. GTA-3 is shown in cross-sectional view in Figure 36 I, and in perspective view in Figure 36 IV (upper right.
    GTA-*4* is a palatal tray useful for anesthetizing any area of the palate, as a preinjection topical, or to eliminate palatal injections. GTA-4 is shown in cross-sectional views in Figure 36 II demonstrating use on the anterior palate (left) and on the posterior palate (right). GTA-4 is shown in perspective view in Figure 36 IV (lower left). GTA-*5* is a mucobuccal tray useful for anesthetizing the mucobuccal fold as a preinjection topical. GTA-5 is shown in cross-sectional views in Figure 36 III demonstrating lower placement (left) and upper placement (right). GTA-5 is shown in perspective view in Figure 36 IV (lower right).

2. Directions for use of GTA-trays
    a. Select appropriate *tray* for area to be anesthetized.
    b. Mix anesthetic: 0.5 ml of 1/1000 Adrenalin[R] (Parke-Davis) to the contents of one 5-ml ampule of 4% lidocaine hydrochloride (4% Xylocaine[R], Astra); dilute to 20 ml with ultrapure water.
    c. Apply Return Electrode (female) to the negative terminal of Phoresor output cable (Fig. 28). If current levels exceed 1.0 mA, it may be necessary to increase the skin electrode area by using 3' × 2' *return electrodes* (GTA 5).
    d. Connect GCE-1 (red *clip electrode*) to GCL-1 (red *clip electrode lead*) and attach to positive *terminal* of the *Phoresor output cable.*
    e. Fill tray with cotton batting so as to surround soft tissue to be anesthetized. GTA-1, 2 and 3 require cotton batting on buccal and lingual. GTA-4 (palatal) requires cotton over the area to be anesthetized. GTA-5 requires cotton in mucobuccal fold. *Note*: in all cases, soaked cotton must touch electrode wire and tissue to be anesthetized. Also, the patient holds GTA-4 and 5 by biting on the occlusal platform. (see Fig. 36 for placement of electrodes).
    f. Apply anesthetic solution to cotton.
    g. Dry teeth; insulate touching metal restorations with soft blue periphery wax (or a suitable substitute).

Diagrams and Placements of GTA-Trays

I, II, III. Cross-sectional Views and
Placement of GTA-Trays
I. GTA-1 (anterior), GTA-2 (small
posterior) or GTA-3 (large
posterior)
II. GTA-4—Palatal tray and
placement (left, anterior
placement; right, posterior
placement)
III. GTA-5—Mucobuccal tray and
placement (left, lower placement;
right upper placement)
IV. Perspective View of GTA Tray Set
(upper l. to r.; GTA 1, 2, 3; lower
l. to r.; GTA 4 and 5)

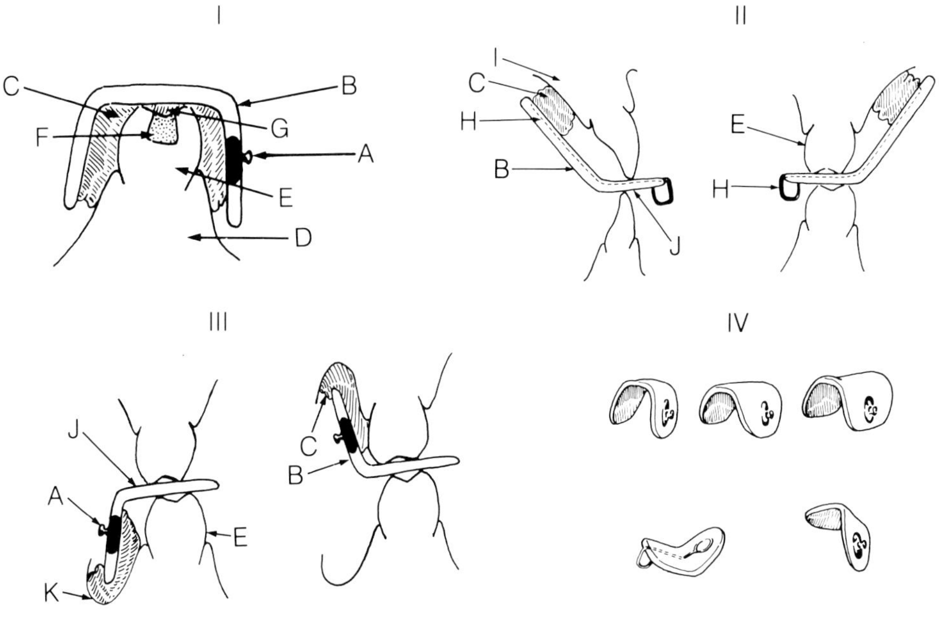

I

II

III

IV

A. Snap (Attach GCE-1)	G. Wax
B. Tray	H. Wire (Attach GCE-1)
C. Cotton	I . Palate
D. Periodontium	J. Occlusal Platform
E. Tooth	K. Mucobuccal Fold
F. Metal Restoration	

Figure 36

h. Insert the *tray* over the teeth and arch, picking up overflow anesthetic with a vacuum. Check for fit of cotton to soft tissue; add more cotton if necessary and re-soak with anesthetic before reinsertion.

i. Reinsert the *tray,* and clip the pre-assembled GCE-1 and GCL-1 (step d.) to the male snap on the tray.

j. Set *Phoresor timer* to past 10 minutes and turn on *current switch.* Slowly adjust current to 1 mA or higher. Then adjust *timer* to deliver 2 mA min. per tooth area (to be anesthetized) as follows:

for:	use:	*mA*	*min*
1 tooth	(GOE-7)	1.0	2
2 tooth	(GTA-1)	1.4	3
3 tooth	(GTA-2)	2.0	3
4 tooth	(GTA-3)	2.0	4

k. Allow about 2 minutes after removal of *tray* for anesthesia to take full effect.

Chapter 15

Instructions for Anti-inflammatory Treatment: Aphthous Ulcer (Canker Sore) or Lichen Planus

Summary

1. Drug—0.125% methylprednisoline sodium succinate (Solu-Medrol^R). Polarity—negative. Some conditions related to use of Solu-Medrol^R are listed in Table 9.
2. *Return electrode*—positive.
Use 1% sodium nitrate as the indifferent electrolyte.
3. Maximum safe current: 0.5 mA for normal size lesions; 1.0 mA for larger areas. Patient threshold and tolerance regulate the amount of current used.
4. Active electrode selection.
Oral electrode with straight-cut large *tip* (GOE-5 or GOE-7).
Large areas—spread cotton over lesion: apply drug to cotton over lesion and to oral electrode.
5. Comments—The author has found two methods useful: (1) the one-step method and (2) the two-step method. In the one-step method, Solu-Medrol^R is applied at the negative electrode. The two-step method involves: first, vasoconstriction and local anesthesia by lidocaine-epinephrine iontophoresis under the positive electrode, then, application of the negative Solu-Medrol^R. The two-step method is used for larger lesions or for highly vascular areas.

One-step Method for Treating Aphthous Ulcers

1. Select drug—Solu-Medrol^R
The powdered drug is prepackaged 25 mg in a capsule. The contents are emptied into 2 ml of ultrapure water in a dappen dish just before use. (The mixed drug deteriorates but can be used for other treatments the same day).
2. Active electrode selection.
Use black *oral electrode* with straight-cut disposable *tip* (GOE-5 or GOE-7)
3. Assembly and placement of *return (skin) electrode* (Fig. 28).
4. Preparation of active electrode.
Snap black *oral electrode* into the *negative terminal* of the *output cable* of the *Phoresor*. Bend flexible *oral electrode* to desired angle for ease of application. Insert *electrode tip* and fill with cotton, leaving it overfilled (2–3 mm). Apply Solu-Medrol^R to the cotton, being certain it is saturated to the metal.
5. Turn the *timer switch* to 10 minutes.
6. Connect active electrode to area of the lesion, making sure that both lesion and borders are covered. If the *plastic tip* is not large enough to cover the entire area, cotton is placed over the lesion, soaked with drug, and the *plastic tip,* applied to the cotton. Slowly turn on the *current switch* until the patient feels a slight tickling sensation in the lesion.

Table 9 Conditions for Treating Oral Lesions

Lesion	Drug	Polarity	How supplied
Inflammatory Example: canker sores (aphthous), lichen planus, or uninfected, traumatic lesions	Solu-Medrol^R (methyl prednisolone sodium succinate)	negative (−)	500 mg powder (Upjohn). Divide powder into 20 doses (#4 Lilly capsules) of 25 mg each. Dilute contents of capsule to 2 ml immediately before use. Shelf life after mixing is 8 hrs.
Viral Example: cold sore (or herpes simplex) lesions or recurrent herpes labialis	Stoxil^R (idoxuridine)	negative (−)	0.1% ophthalmic solution keep refrigerated; observe drug shelf life.
Bacterial Example: infected wounds or sores	tetracycline HCl	Positive	125 mg capsules; use ½ of powder from a capsule diluted to 20 ml with ultrapure water
	clindamycin phosphate	negative	use Cleocin T^R, Topical solution (1% clindamycin phosphate)

Aphthous lesions are quite sensitive and most of them are treated at 0.2—0.5 mA. Adjust current downward to eliminate uncomfortable sensation.

7. Current maximum—0.5 mA or patient threshold.

8. Adjust the *timer switch* to appropriate number of minutes as follows:

mA	min
0.2	10
0.3	7
0.4	5
0.5	4

The assistant can hold the electrode for the dentist, allowing him to perform other work. Evacuation may be necessary to control saliva.

9. At the end of treatment, remove electrodes and evaluate. There will usually be a tingling sensation for 2-3 minutes after removing the electrode; the patient should experience relief of discomfort after 3-5 minutes and rapid healing during the next 2-4 days. A second treatment is rarely needed.

Two-step Method (used for larger lesions or those in highly vascular areas).

1. Step 1. Local anesthesia and vasoconstriction.

a. Apply lidocaine ointment to the lesion while preparing drugs and electrodes.

b. Select drug—1% lidocaine with 1/40,000 epinephrine or Xylocaine[R] green-coded cartridges. The Solu-Medrol[R], for step two, can be mixed at this time (see above).

c. Active electrode selection—red *oral electrode* with straight—cut *plastic tip* (GOE-5 or 7).

d. Assembly and placement of *return* (skin) *electrode* (Fig. 28).

e. Preparation of active electrode. Snap red *oral electrode* into *output cable* of the Phoresor. Bend flexible *oral electrode* to desired angle for ease of application. Insert straight—cut *plastic tip* and fill with cotton, leaving it somewhat overfilled. Apply lidocaine-epinephrine solution to the cotton being certain that the solution saturating the cotton touches the metal tip of the oral electrode.

f. Set *timer switch* to more than 10 minutes.

g. Apply electrode to lesion using 0.2 mA for 5 min, 0.3 mA for 4 min, 0.4 mA for 3 min or 0.5 mA for 2 min. (Total dose: 1.0 mA-min.)

2. Step 2. Solu-Medrol[R] Treatment.
Follow all procedures for one-step method of aphthous ulcer treatment (see pages 127, 128). The one-step method is used on smaller ulcers in the anterior portion of the vestibule. The two-step method is used in the posterior vestibule in the floor of the mouth or on large lesions.

Treatment of Lichen Planus

The treatment of lichen planus is the same as the one-step method for aphthous ulcer treatment (see above) except that a larger electrode is usually needed to cover the lesion, a higher current level is used and repeat treatments are often needed. The lesion is dried and a layer of cotton is placed so that the lesion is covered. The cotton, both over the lesion and in the electrode tip, is soaked with Solu-Medrol[R]. The *oral electrode* is placed against the cotton covering the lesion; current is applied for 2 mA-min. per cm^2; This is repeated three times over a period of a week. The lesion should then be more comfortable, with no evidence of inflammation or erosive process.

Systemic factors should be considered as part of the treatment. If a relapse occurs, the treatments can be repeated every 3-6 months.

Before the Solu-Medrol[R] iontophoresis is performed, the patient's general health and all local and systemic factors are considered. Any factor which requires correction is performed in order to bring the patient to the best state of oral and systemic health.

Chapter 16

Instructions for Antiviral Therapy

Summary

1. Drug–Stoxil[R] (idoxuridine, 0.1%, ophthalmic solution) Polarity–negative. Some conditions related to use of Stoxil[R] are listed in Table 9).
2. Return electrode–positive (GRE-4). Use 1% sodium nitrate as the indifferent electrolyte (see Fig. 28).
3. Active electrode. Black *oral electrode* (GOE-2) with straight cut; *plastic tip* (GOE-5 or 7).
4. Maximum current. Minimum lesion size–0.5 mA; larger lesions; 1.0 mA.
5. Specific *Contraindications* for Stoxil[R] Iontophoresis are:
   a. pregnancy,
   b. simple lesions which remain small, occur infrequently and heal uneventfully,
   c. viral resistance to idoxuridine, and
   d. allergy to idoxuridine.
6. Specific *Indications* for Stoxil[R] Iontophoresis are:
   a. History of spread of lesions to other parts of the body, especially the eye,
   b. To prevent spread of infections in persons who are liable to have a disastrous generalized herpes infection, such as: (1) small infants, treat the primary attack and protect the infant by treating recurrent attacks in parents and nursery workers; and (2) immune compromised persons, treat the herpes lesions and protect the patient by treating recurrent attacks in family members and in hospital personnel.
   c. Massive recurrent attack involving one-fourth or more of the lips and generally interfering with alimentation, speech and appearance.
   d. Interference with one's profession, such as that of a speaker or a wind-instrument player.
   e. A primary attack.

Treatment

The procedures for treatment of herpes simplex infections are the same as for aphthous ulcer treatment (one-step method) except for drug selection.
1. Drug selection–Stoxil[R] (idoxuridine, 0.1% ophthalmic solution). Obtain this from the pharmacist and use undiluted. Polarity is negative.
2. Follow all succeeding procedures (2–8) for aphthous ulcer treatment, except for substitution of Stoxil[R] for Solu-Medrol[R] (see Chapter 15).

Results

Coalescence of vesicles, increased rate of oozing, lack of spread of lesions and rapid healing. Rarely, a second treatment is needed (see pages 39–45).

Chapter 17

Miscellaneous Considerations

Sterilization Procedure

The active electrodes and other non-disposable items used should be first cleaned and then sterilized, by soaking the part, in Cidex^R (glutaraldehyde) for at least 20 minutes. Follow the manufacturer's directions for mixing and handling Cidex^R. Rinse all objects, removing Cidex^R before handling, as Cidex^R is irritating and caustic. Cidex^R has a broad spectrum of antimicrobial activity.

Electrodes should never be "flamed" or autoclaved, as the flexible vinyl material will not withstand high temperatures.

Wipe all other parts with alcohol after use. Iontophoresis can be performed on healthy patients without aseptic technique using normal precautions for cleanliness. Dispose plastic tips after 1 or 2 uses.

Unusual cases, such as severe diabetics or immune-compromised patients, may require additional precautions for sterilization and asepsis. *Caution:* Electrodes are for external use only. Since the electrode parts are not sterile they should not be applied to open wounds without further disinfection.

Device Controlled by Medical Device Amendments of 1976

The ElectroApplicator System is a device controlled by the Medical Device Amendments of 1976 and the following should be observed.

Caution: Federal Law (U.S.A.) restricts this device to use on order of a physician or dentist.

Warnings: For external use only. Not recommended to be used for patients with known myocardial disease or arrhythmias without advice of a physician. Do not use on open wounds. If a patient experiences discomfort during the treatment, disconnect the patient; check all systems before reconnecting.

Precautions: Avoid discomfort by slowly increasing the *current switch* while operating the iontophoresor, and by returning the *current switch* to zero before reconnecting or connecting the patient to the iontophoresor. If the patient is uncomfortable during the treatment, this may indicate that too much current is being applied. An excess of direct current may cause a burn. Observe preset limits of current and do not exceed patient tolerance.

The ElectroApplicator System should be used only with the parts described and according to the Instruction Manual supplied with the system. Any alterations by the dentist are at his own discretion.

Contraindications: There are no known absolute contraindications unless a patient is allergic to the drug being used. The only *relative* contraindication is for use in a patient with cardiac disease.

Side Effects: There is often a transient erythema at the site of the return electrode. This disappears shortly after removal of the electrode.

Contraindications

The only relative contraindication for the use of iontophoresis is for use in a patient with cardiac arrythmia or a cardiac pacemaker. Application of electrical devices to these patients might present a hazardous situation. However, the amount of current applied during iontophoresis is negligible. The battery operated Phoresor™ should present *no* safety hazard to any patient because the patient is never connected to the electrical line-circuit. Nevertheless, the heart patient might construe the application of an iontophoresor as a hazard, especially if a coincidental accident happens. Physician evaluation is advised; if the dentist feels he should treat such a patient with the iontophoresor, a release form should be obtained from the patient. A sample of a release form is shown in Figure 37.

Warranty and Service

The Phoresor™ is warranted against defects in its manufacture by Motion Control, Inc. and by Dentelect Corp. for a period of one year from the date of its purchase. If under normal use, the unit should fail during this period, Motion Control, Inc. (at its option) will either repair or replace the defective unit. If it should become necessary to return your unit for service, please ship the Phoresor™ to:

Dentelect Corporation
Box 4565
Augusta, Georgia 30907
Phone: (404) 738-7511

Dentelect Corp. is responsible for quality and workmanship of the Dentelect Electrode Set™ by LPG. In case of a complaint concerning any component of the Dentelect Electrode Set™, please contact Dentelect as described above.

Repaired or replaced units, or components, will be returned by UPS. The customer is responsible for all shipping charges. Please check all components before returning for repairs.

Checking the EAS before Operation

Before operation is attempted, the dentist should use the following steps to assure correct operation of the system.

1. Insert battery. Slide battery compartment door at rear of *Phoresor* to *open* position, insert battery and close door. If battery is *improperly* inserted, a constant audible signal will be noted. Always keep a spare fresh battery available and replace battery, whenever the battery reject light comes on.
2. Turn *current switch on*—This causes a reject signal because the *timer* must be turned on first (return *current switch* to *off* after each reject).
3. Turn Timer to past 5 min and turn *on current switch*. A double zero should enter on the dosage current display. Gradually turn up *current switch* until a reject occurs. This position of the *current switch* should be noted as the *true zero* which usually occurs between 9 and 3 o'clock on the dial: The *true zero* is important because it is the point at which current is first delivered, a safety feature which prevents a surge of current into the patient. The reject after the *true zero* signals that the external circuit is not connected.
4. Connect the external circuit with a 5000

**Release Form for
Iontophoresis on a Heart Patient**

I _____ wish to have my teeth or mouth

treated by iontophoresis as explained by my dentist, Dr. _____.
Although I have a heart condition, I understand that connecting this battery operated device to me is safe in all respects and that the device does not generate
enough current to cause any damage to my heart when applied from the exterior

of my body. This has been explained to my physician, Dr. _____
and he agrees that the treatment can cause me no harm. I therefore grant permission to have iontophoresis used on my teeth or mouth.

Signed: _____

Date: _____

Witnessed by:

_____ Dr. _____ D.D.S.

(Multiple copies of this page may be made without permission of the Author or Publisher)

Fig. 37   Release form for cardiac patient.

ohm resistor (part G-5000). (If G-5000 is missing, notify Dentelect so that it can be supplied to you.) Now turn on the *current switch* and gradually increase to the *true zero* you should notice an mA reading; continue increasing to the maximum reading (2.0 mA ± 0.1). If a reject occurs with G-5000 connected, then the Phoresor should be returned to Dentelect for repairs. (*Note:* There must be no breaks in G-5000.)

5. Check each lead of the DES-1 as follows:
   a. Connect the black *oral electrode* (GOE-2) to the Phoresor; the metal end of GOE-2 should touch G-5000, which is connected to the red terminal of the Phoresor output cable. You should obtain a full reading, with no reject upon maximum increase of the *current switch.*
   b. Fill the *brush electrode* (GBE-2) reservoir with NaF, connect to GOE-2, soak bristles in NaF solution and repeat steps in a. above, except contact bristles of GBE-2 to G-5000.
   c. Connect black *clip electrode lead* (GCL-2) to *clip electrode* (GCE-2) and repeat step a. above, except connect clip to G-5000.
   d. Switch G-5000 to negative terminal of output cable and check all red connections as described above; a., check GOE-1, b., check GBE-2 (GBE-1 has been omitted), and c., check GCL-1 and GCE-1.

Loose connections in these leads will cause rejects. If you have any unusable leads, return them to Dentelect and they will be replaced.

Trouble Shooting the ElectroApplicator System (EAS) Model-2

In use of the EAS, an occasional problem arises which will result in a reject by the Phoresor. Although this may be a source of annoyance, the reject feature actually helps us to perform iontophoresis safely, effectively and comfortably for the patient. The reject warns us when something is faulty. The following will help you to find the cause of the reject.

There are three types of rejects:

Type I. (Formerly *Type A) Battery reject—yellow light on.
Type II. (Formerly *Type C) Reject at position (6 o'clock).
Type III. (Formerly *Type B) Reject at True zero (9 to 3 o'clock).

Table 10 is a Troubleshooting Chart showing types of rejects and their correction. Rejects should be checked in the order presented in Table 10.

*Instruction Manual, EAS, Model C-2, Feb. 1980, Dentelect Corp., Augusta, GA

Table 10   Troubleshooting Chart (check in order presented)

Type	#	Description	Causes	Remedy
I.	I.1	Battery reject (yellow light)	Low battery	Replace battery at rear of unit. Purchase a spare battery as soon as possible.
II.	II.1	TIMER	TIMER not on	Turn timer past 5 minutes before any treatment is started.
	II.2	Defective Phoresor	Improper internal connection(s)	Check with Part G-5000. Return defective Phoresor to Dentelect Corp.
	II.3[†]	Polarization of skin	Skin acts as a battery. (This occurs in some patients or sometimes after multiple treatments).	Determine if current will flow in skin by holding Active Electrode against nearby skin area. If current will not flow, replace Skin Electrode (II.3) to nearby site or replace Skin Electrode to other arm.
III.	III.1	Electrode	Poor connection(s)	Recheck all connection(s) before restart. Check lead wires for signs of wearing or fraying. Make sure pad of Skin Electrode is soaked with $NaNO_3$ and is flat against the skin. Cotton in plastic tip must be soaked to the metal, and have no air spaces between pieces of cotton. Brush reservoir must be filled and bristles soaked. Clip electrode must be securely fastened to tray handle and banana plug must be securely inserted into other end.
	III.2	Metal not insulated	Low resistance	Be certain that all metal restorations are covered with blue periphery wax or two coats of Copalite[R].
	III.3	Defective skin electrode	Contact of metal to pad	Replace with a new Skin Electrode.* Wipe skin with alcohol.
Other		Treatment completed	End of treatment	Turn *off* current switch

*Dentelect Corp. will gladly replace any defective Skin Electrodes which are used to check this step.
[†]Polarization is a type II reject but it is checked after III.3.

References

1. Abell, E. and Morgan, K.: The treatment of idiopathic hyperhidrosis by glycopyrronium bromide and tap water iontophoresis. Br. J. Dermatol., 91: 87–91, 1974.
2. Abramowitsch, D., and Neoussikine, B.: *Treatment by Ion Transfer (Iontophoresis),* Grune and Stratton, New York, 1976. 186 pp.
3. *Accepted Dental Therapeutics,* 37th edition, American Dental Association, Chicago, IL. 1977, p. 113.
4. Adriani, J. and Campbell, D.: Fatalities following topical application of local anesthetics to mucous membranes. JAMA 162: 1527–1530, 1956.
5. Benedicenti, A., and Cingano, L., eds. Manual of iontophoresis in the oral cavity (Drug electrophoresis in stomatology) [in Italian]. Scuola Tipografica del Sorriso Francescano, Genoa. 88 pp.
6. Boone, D. C.: Hyaluronidase iontophoresis. Physical Therapy, 49: 139–145, 1969.
7. Brännström, M., and Nyborg, H.: Pulp reaction to fluoride solution applied to deep cavities. An experimental histologial study. J. Dent. Res. 50: 1548–1552, 1971.
8. Brännström, M. and Aström, A.: The hydrodynamics of the dentin: Its possible relationship to dentinal pain. Int. Dent. J. 22: 219–227, 1972.
9. Chasens, A. I. and Kaslick, R. S. (Editors): Mechanisms of pain and sensitivity in the teeth and supporting tissues: A workshop presented by Fairleigh Dickinson University and the American Academy of Oral Medicine, Nov. 12–13, 1973. Fairleigh Dickinson Univ., 1974.
10. Collins, E. M.: Desensitization of hypersensitive teeth. Dent. Dig. 68: 360–363, 1962.
11. Comeau, M., Brummett, R., and Vernon, J.: Local anesthesia of the ear by iontophoresis. Arch. Otolaryngol 98: 114–120, 1973.
12. Echols, F., Norris, C. H., and Tabb, H. G.: Anesthesia of the ear by iontophoresis of lidocaine. Arch Otolaryngol. 101: 418–421, 1975.
13. Ehrlich, J., Hochman, N., Gedalia, I. and Tal, M.: Residual fluoride concentration and scanning electron microscopic examination of root surfaces of human teeth after topical application of fluoride *in vivo.* J. Dent. Res. 54: 897–900, 1975.
14. Eshleman, J. R. and Leonard, E. D., Jr.: Desensitization of dentin by iontophoresis: A review and case reports: J. Oral Therap. Pharmacol. 1:526, 1965.
15. Fellner, R., and Glawogger, F.: Penicillin -iontophorese in der augenheilkunde. Klin. Montasbl. Augenheilk, 160: 300–303, 1972.
16. Gangarosa, L. P.: Iontophoresis for surface local anesthesia. JADA, 88: 125–128, 1974.
17. Walton, R., Gangarosa, L. P., Leonard, L., Sharawy, M.: Pulp and dentin response to iontophoresis of NaF on exposed roots, J. Dent. Res. 55: B228, #667, 1976.
18. Gangarosa, L. P., Merchant, H. W., Park, N. H., and Hill, J. M.: Iontophoretic application of idoxuridine for recurrent herpes labialis. Presented at AADR Meeting, J. Dent. Res. #569, 1977a.
19. Gangarosa, L. P., Park, N. H., and Hill, J. M.: Iontophoretic assistance of 5-iodo-2'-deoxuridine penetration into neonatal mouse skin and effects on DNA synthesis. Proc. Soc. Exp. Biol. Med. 154: 439–443, 1977b.
20. Park, N. H., Gangarosa, L. P., and Hill, J. M.: Iontophoretic application of Ara-AMP (9-β-D-arabinofuranosyladenine- 5' -monophosphate) into adult mouse skin. Proc. Soc. Exp. Biol. Med. 156: 326–329, 1977c.

21. Hill, J. M., Gangarosa, L. P., and Park, N. H.: Iontophoretic application of antiviral chemotherapeutic agents. Ann. of N.Y. Acad. of Sci. 284: 604–612, 1977d.

22. Gangarosa, L. P., Park, N. H. and King, G: Iontophoresis of lidocaine into frog sciatic nerve fibers. Life Sciences, 21: 885–890, 1977e.

23. Park, N. H., Gangarosa, L. P., Kwon, B., and Hill, J. M.: Iontophoretic application of adenine arabinoside monophosphate (Ara-AMP) to HSV-1 infected hairless mouse skin. Antimicrob. Agents Chemother. 14(4): 605–608, 1978a.

24. Gangarosa, L. P., and Park, N. H.: Practical considerations in iontophoresis of fluoride for desensitizing dentin. J. of Pros. Dent. 39(2): 173–178, 1978b.

25. Gangarosa, L. P., Heuer, G. A., Park, N. H., Hayes, B. B., Little, C. K., Baker, G. W. and Smith, M. A.: Desensitizing hypersensitive dentin by iontophoresis with fluoride. NYS Dent. J. 44(3): 92–94, 1978c.

26. Gangarosa, L. P., Robertson, E., Park, N. H., Parker, R. L., and Hayes, B. B.: Defining the ideal local anesthetic solution for iontophoresis. Presented at IADR meeting, J. Dent. Res., 57: 119, #180, 1978d.

27. Gangarosa, L. P., Park, N. H., Fong, B. C., Scott, D. F., and Hill, J. M: Conductivity of drugs used for iontophoresis. J. of Pharm. Sci. 67(10): 1439–1443, 1978e.

28. Gangarosa, L. P., Merchant, H. W., Park, N. H. and Hill, J. M.: Iontophoretic application of idoxuridine for recurrent herpes labialis. Report of preliminary clinical trials. Meth. and Find. Exptl. Clin. Pharmacol.: 105–109, 1979a.

29. Kwon, B. S., Hill, J. M., Wiggins, C., Tuggle, C., and Gangarosa, L. P.: Iontophoretic application of adenine arabinoside monophosphate for the treatment of herpes simplex virus type 2 skin infections in hairless mice. J. of Infect. Des. 140, 1014, 1979b.

30. Walton, R. E., Leonard, L. A., Sharawy, M., and Gangarosa, L. P.: Effects on pulp of iontophoresis of sodium fluoride on exposed roots in dogs. Oral Surg. 48(6): 545–557, 1979c.

31. Gibson, L. E., and Cooke, R. E.: A test for concentration of electrolytes in sweat in cystic fibrosis of the pancreas utilizing pilocarpine by iontophoresis. Pediatrics 23: 545–549, 1959.

32. Goodman, L. S., and Gilman, A. (eds.): The Pharmacological Basis of Therapeutics, 5th edition; Macmillan Publishing Co., Inc., New York; 1975, p. 1051.

33. Gordon, B. I. and Maibach, H. I.: Eccrine anhidrosis to glutaraldehyde formaldehyde and iontophoresis. J. Invest. Derm. 53: (6), 436–439, 1969.

34. Gordon, A. H. and Weinstein, M. V.: Sodium salicylate iontophoresis in the treatment of plantar warts. Phys. Ther. 49(8): 869–870, 1969.

35. Graykowski, E. and Holroyd, S. W.: Therapeutic management of primary herpes, recurrent labial herpes, aphthous stomatitis and Vincent's infection. Dent. Clin. of N. A., 14(4): 721–731, 1970.

36. Greminger, R. F., Elliott, Jr., R. A., and Rapperport, A.: Antibiotic iontophoresis for the management of burned ear chondritis. Plast. Reconstr. Surg. 66:356–359, 1980.

37. Grice, K. A. and Bettley, F. R.: Inhibition of sweating by poldine methosulphate (Nacton), Brit. J. Derm. 78: 458–464, 1966.

38. Grice, K. A., Sattar, H. and Baker, H.: Treatment of idiopathic hyperhydrosis with iontophoresis of tap water and poldine methosulphate. Br. J. Derm. 86: 72–78, 1972.

39. Grossman, L: A systematic method for the treatment of hypersensitive dentin. J. Am. Dent. Assoc. 22: 592–602, 1931.

40. Harris, R.: Iontophoresis, Ch. 4 in Therapeutic Electricity and Ultraviolet Radiation. pp. 156–178, Sidney Licht (Ed.), E. Licht (Publisher), Baltimore, 1959, (Reprinted in 2nd ed., 1967)

41. Hayasaki, K., Kitamura, T., and Kaneko, T.: Application of BLM-iontophoresis for the tumor-therapy of the head and neck area. J. Jap. Soc. Cancer Ther. 12(4): 522–527, 1977.

42. Hiatt, W. H. and Johansen, E.: Root preparation. I. Obturation of dentinal tubules in treatment of root hypersensitivity. J. Periodont. 43: 373–380, 1972.

43. Hoyt, W. H. and Bibby, B. G.: Use of sodium fluoride for desensitizing dentin, J. Am. Dent. Assoc. 30: 1372, 1943.

44. Hyndiuk, R. A., Hull, D. S., Schultz, R. O., Chin, G. N., Laibson, P. R. and Krachmer, J. H.: Adenine arabinoside in idoxuridine unresponsive and intolerant herpetic keratitis. Am. J. Ophthalmol. 79: 655–658, 1975.

45. Iontophoresis—A major advancement. (Editorial), Eye, Ear, Nose & Throat, 55: 41–42, L976(2), 1976.

46. Itoi, M., Gefter, J. W., Kaneko, N., Ishii, Y., Ramer, R. M., and Gasset, A. R.: Teratogenicities of ophthalmic drugs I. Antiviral ophthalmic drugs. Arch. Ophthalmol. 93: 46–51, 1975.

47. Jacobsen, S. and Stephen, R.: Drugs delivered without a needle via ionization. Med. News & Int. Report: p.1, Mar. 6, 1978.

48. Jenkinson, D. M., and McLean, J. A.: The potential use of iontophoresis in the treatment of skin disorders. Vet. Rec., 94: 8–12, 1974.

49. Jensen, A. L.: Hypersensitivity controlled by iontophoresis: double-blind clinical investigation. J. Am. Dent. Assoc. 86: 216–225, 1964.

50. Johnson, G. and Brännström, M.: The sensitivity of dentin. Changes in relation to conditions at exposed tubule apertures. Acta. Odont. Scand. 32: 29–38, 1974.

51. Kahn, J.: Calcium iontophoresis in suspected myopathy. Phys. Ther., 55(4): 476–477, 1975.

52. Kahn, J.: Acetic acid iontophoresis for calcium deposits, Phys. Ther., 57(6): 658–659, 1977.

53. Kanai, M., and Maruyama, Y.: Over-all study concerning ion permeation in the hard tissues of the tooth, J. Oral Science Assoc. 13, 1954.

54. Kanai, M.: Device for penetrating teeth with fluoride 1958, United States Patent #2834344.

55. Kaufman, H. E.: Clinical cure for herpes simplex keratitis by 5-iodo-2'-deoxyuridine. Proc. Soc. Expt. Biol. Med. 109: 251–252, 1961.

56. LaForest, N. R. and Cofrancesco, C.: Antibiotic iontophoresis in the treatment of ear chondritis. Phys. Ther. 58(1), 32–34, 1978.

57. Leduc, S.: Electric Ions and Their Use in Medicine. Rebman Ltd., London, 1908.

58. Lefkowitz, W., and Bodecker, C. F.: Sodium fluoride: Its effect on the dental pulp. Ann. Dent. 3: 141, 1945.

59. Lefkowitz, W.: Pulp response to ionization. J. Prosthet. Dent. 12: 966–976, 1962.

60. Lefkowitz, W., Burdick, H. D., and Moore, D. L.: Desensitization of dentin by bioelectric induction of secondary dentin. J. Pros. Dent. 13: 940–949, 1963.

61. Levit, F.: Simple device for treatment of hyperhidrosis by iontophoresis. Arch. Derm., 98: 505–507, 1968.

62. Leyden, J. J.: Disorders of the Mouth in Conn's Current Therapy, H. F. Conn (Ed.), W. B. Saunders Co., 1975, p. 596–599.

63. Lukomsky, E. H.: Fluorine therapy for exposed dentin and alveolar atrophy. J. Dent. Res. 20: 649–658, 1941.

64. Machen, J. B., and Johnson, R.: Desensitization model learning and the dental behavior of children. J. Dent. Res. 53: 83–87, 1974.

65. Manning M. M.: New approach to desensitization of cervical dentin. Dent. Survey. 37: 731, 1961.

66. Maurice, C. G. and Schour, I.: Effects of sodium fluoride upon the pulp of the rat molar. J. Dent. Res. 35: 69, 1956.

67. Meffert, R. M., and Hoskins, S. W.: Effect of a strontium chloride dentifrice in relieving dental hypersensitivity. J. Periodont., 35: 232, 1964.

68. Minkov, B., Marmari, L., Gedalia, E., and Garfunkel, A.: The effectiveness of sodium fluoride treatment with and without iontophoresis on the reduction of hypersensitive dentin. J. Periodontol. 46: 246, 1975.

69. Moawad, M. B.: Treatment of vitiligo with 1% solution of the sodium salt of meladinine using the iontophoresis technique. Derm. Mschr. 155: 388–394, 1969.

70. Morton, W. J.: Guaiacol-cocain cataphoresis and local anesthesia: A new cataphoresis electrode and the Wheeler fractional volt selector. The Dental Cosmos, 38: 48–53, 1896.

71. Murthy, K. S., Talim, S. T., and Singh, I.: A comparative evaluation of topical application and iontophoresis of sodium fluoride for desensitization of hypersensitive dentin. Oral surg. 36: 448–458, 1973.

72. Nahmias, A. J. and Roizman, B.: Infection with herpes-simplex virus 1 and 2 (three parts). N. Engl. J. Med. 289: 667–674, 719–725, 781–789, 1973.

73. O'Malley, E. P. and Oester, Y. T.: Influence of some physical chemical factors of iontophoresis using radio-isotopes. Arch. Phys. Med. & Rehab. 36: 310–316, 1955.

74. Pashley, D. H., Livingston, M. J., Reeder, O. W. and Horner, J.: Effects of the degree of tubule occlusion on the permeability of human dentin in vitro. Arch. Oral Biol. 23: 1127–1133, 1979.

75. Peterson, B. E. and Strelkova, R. M.: Ad-

ministration of antitumor preparations by electrophoresis. Vepresy Otologli. 10(6): 545–547, 1965.

76. *Physician's Desk Reference,* 32 edition, Pub. Charles, E. Baker, Jr. Medical Economics Co., Oradell, N. J., 1978.

77. Prusoff, W. H. and Goz, B.: Potential mechanisms of action of antiviral agents. Fed. Proc. 32: 1679–1689, 1973.

78. Pusso-Carrasco, H.: Strontium chloride toothpaste-effectiveness as related to duration of use. Pharmacol. Ther. Dent. 1: 209–215, 1971.

79. Ross, M. R.: Hypersensitive teeth: Effect of strontium chloride in a compatible dentifrice. J. Periodont. 32: 49, 1961.

80. Rothfeld, S. H., and Murray, W.: The treatment of Peyronie's disease by iontophoresis of C_{21} esterfied glucocorticoids. J. of Urology, 97: 874–875, 1967.

81. Rovelstad, G. H., and St. John, W. E.: The condition of the young dental pulp after the application of sodium fluoride to freshly cut dentin. J. Am. Dent. Assoc. 39: 670–682, 1949.

82. Schaeffer, M. L., Bixler, D., and Yu, P. L.: The effectiveness of iontophoresis in reducing cervical hypersensitivity. J. Periodontol. 42: 695–700, 1971.

83. Scott, H. M., Jr.: Reduction of sensitivity by electrophoresis. J. Dent. Child 29: 225–241, 1962.

84. Seltzer, S.: *Pain Control in Dentistry: Diagnosis and Management,* J. B. Lippincott Co., Philadelphia and Toronto, 1978.

85. Shelley, W. B., Horvath, P. N., Weidman, F. D. and Pillsbury, D. M.: Production of sweat retention anhidrosis and vesicles by means of iontophoresis. J. Invest. Derm. 11: 275–291, 1948.

86. Shelley, W. B., and Horvath, P. N.: Experimental miliaria in man: II. Production of sweat retention anhidrosis and miliaria crystallina by various kinds of injury. J. Invest. Derm. 14: 9–20, 1960.

87. Shrivastava, S. N. and Singh, G.: Tap water iontophoresis in palmoplantar hyperhidrosis. Br. J. Derm., 96, 189–195, 1977.

88. Siemon, W. H.: A new approach in solving the problem of hypersensitivity and postoperative distress in dentin and cementum. J. Conn. State Dent. Assoc. 34: 5–10, 1960.

89. Simor, G. G.: Toothbrush for producing electrical potentials. U.S. Patent #3478741, 1969.

90. Sisler, H. A.: Iontophoretic local anesthesia for conjunctival surgery. Annals of Ophthal., 10(5): 597–598, 1978.

91. Souder, W., and Schoonover, I. C.: Experimental remineralization of dentin. J. Am. Dent. Assoc. 31: 1579–1586, 1944.

92. Stanley, H. R., White, C. L., and McCray, L.: The rate of tertiary (reparative) dentin formation in the human tooth. Oral Surg. 21: 579–589, 1966.

93. Stone, T. W.: Responses of blood vessels to various amines applied by microiontophoresis. J. Pharm. Pharmacol. 24: 318–323, 1972.

94. von Sallmann, L.: Sulfadiazine iontophoresis in pyocyaneus infection of rabbit cornea. Am. J. Ophthal. 25: 1292–1300, 1942.

95. von Sallmann, L.: Penetration of penicillin into the eye. Arch. Ophthal. 34, 195–201, 1945.

96. Weir, C. D.: Intranasal ionization in the treatment of vasomotor nasal disorders. J. Laryngol., 81: 1143–1150, 1967.

97. Wilson, J. M., B. W. Fry, R. E. Walton, and L. P. Gangarosa, Sr.: Fluoride levels in dentin after iontophoresis of 2% NaF. J. Dent. Res. 60A:462, #609, 1981.

98. Witzcl, S. H., Fielding, I. Z., and Ormsby, H. L.: Ocular penetration of antibiotics by iontophoresis. J. Ophthal. 42: 89–95, 1956.

Practice and Science in Dentistry

quintessence
books

Henry M. Goldman, D.M.D./
Alan M. Shuman, D.M.D./Gerald A. Isenberg, D.D.S.

An Atlas of the Surgical
Management of Periodontal Disease

The purpose of this new atlas is to acquaint clinicians with current surgical techniques in the treatment of periodontal disease. Basic operations that have proven successful are reviewed with concise, sequential explanations. The numerous color illustrations were carefully selected to depict classic cases as well as the results of treatment. An excellent introductory or review text.

224 pages; 403 illustrations (351 color)
Linen-bound with dust cover; 17.5 x 24.5 cm
ISBN 0-931386-41-1

Published 1982

Herbert T. Shillingburg, Jr., D.D.S./James C. Kessler, B.S., D.D.S.

Restoration of the Endodontically Treated Tooth

Endodontic therapy has spread within the dental profession. Teeth that were once extracted are now saved. But treatment is not complete until the tooth has been restored to complete function in a cosmetically acceptable way. The present text identifies principles of endodontic restoration and describes fourteen specific ways of rebuilding an endodontically treated tooth for subsequent restoration. Step-by-step explanations and clear illustrations make this an essential guide for the novice and a practical reference for the experienced clinician.

374 pages; 739 illustrations (231 color)
Linen-bound with dust cover; 17.5 x 24.5 cm
ISBN 0-87615-108-0

Published 1982

Practice and Science in Dentistry

quintessence
books

Diarmuid B. Shanley
Division of Periodontology, Trinity College, Dublin University

Efficacy of Treatment Procedures in Periodontics

*"A must as a reference book to teachers, graduate students and
all practising periodontists."*
Journal of the Canadian Dental Association

Proceedings of a workshop held at Trinity College, Dublin. International experts discuss plaque control as a realistic community objective, as well as efficacy of periodontal surgical procedures, pathology of periodontal diseases, and the establishment of priorities. An excellent reference for practitioner and student alike.

344 pages; 48 illustrations
Linen-bound with dust cover; 17.5 x 24.5 cm
ISBN 0-931386-43-8

Published 1980

Fermin A. Carranza, Jr., Dr. Odont./E. Barrie Kenney, D.D.S., M.S.
Section of Periodontology, School of Dentistry
University of California, Los Angeles

Prevention of Periodontal Disease

Preeminent in these proceedings was the promotion of dialogue among periodontal authorities to identify a philosophical basis as well as specific technical aspects of prevention. Leading periodontists explore such modalities as pulsating water lavage, nutrition counseling, and behavior modification, in addition to reviewing the specific plaque hypothesis and clinical research. A necessary addition to your library.

100 pages
Washable cover; 17.5 x 24.5 cm
ISBN 0-931386-51-9

Published 1981